JUNK SCIENCE JUDO

JUNK SCIENCE JUDO

SELF-DEFENSE AGAINST
HEALTH SCARES & SCAMS

STEVEN J. MILLOY

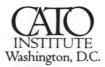

CATO INSTITUTE
Washington, D.C.

Library of Congress Cataloging-in-Publication Data

Milloy, Steven J.
  Junk science judo : self-defense against health scares and scams / by Steven J.
    Milloy. p. cm.
  Includes bibliographical references and index.
  ISBN 1-930865-12-0
    1. Quacks and quackery. 2. Consumer education. 3. Fraud—
Prevention. 4. Consumer protection. I. Title.

R730 .M554 2001
615.8'56—dc21

                                                                    2001042430

Cover design by Amanda Elliott.

Printed in the United States of America.

CATO INSTITUTE
1000 Massachusetts Ave., N.W.

To my daughter Ali:

Seek the truth.

It will set you free.

CONTENTS

PREFACE

IN THE DARK DAYS before April Fool's Day 1996, the junk science crowd marauded with impunity. Dastardly rogues freely deceived a hapless public with bogus science to advance their own special and misanthropic interests. Then, JunkScience.com was born.

More than five years and millions of JunkScience.com visitors later, the Junksters remain largely untouchable. Well, not all of them. One notorious scoundrel went down hard—courtesy of JunkScience.com. By January 1999, Dr. George Lundberg had been the editor of the prestigious *Journal of the American Medical Association* for 17 years. Lundberg had often abused his position as editor of *JAMA* to publish unabashed junk science.

Lundberg understandably advocated against smoking. But he allowed his advocacy to cloud his scientific judgment. Lundberg once published a study in *JAMA* reporting that secondhand smoke caused hearing problems—supposedly more than smoking.[1] This is somewhat counterintuitive since smokers are exposed to their own secondhand smoke and, therefore, should have a much greater risk of hearing problems—that is, if the theory had any merit at all. Certainly excessive smoking increases the risk of numerous diseases. But that didn't justify publishing such a bizarre study.

Lundberg published a study in *JAMA* reporting that in states with felony laws requiring safe gun storage, accidental deaths of children by gunfire dropped by more than 40 percent.[2] But the study was fatally flawed. The researchers did not collect any data indicating that compliance with safe storage laws was the cause of the reduction in gun accidents. They merely assumed a cause-and-effect relationship based on a weak and unreliable statistical correlation between safe storage laws and gun accident rates.

Lundberg ignored this glaring weakness and timed publication of the study to coincide with the campaign for Initiative 676 in Washington State, a provision that would, among other things, require trigger locks on all handguns sold or transferred.

And consider this report on Lundberg from the *New York Times Magazine*:

> On a dreary Monday several months ago, . . . Dr. George Lundberg, editor of the Journal of the American Medical Association, stretched across the clutter in his sprawling corner office to confide his latest coup. The lead article in next week's issue, "Fish Consumption and Risk of Sudden Cardiac Death," was, he murmured, "really hot." A steely-eyed pathologist with a finely honed news sense, Lundberg is rarely wrong on such matters, in part because he leaves nothing to chance.
>
> The previous Tuesday, the American Medical Association press office deluged 2,500 media outlets around the world with press packets, E-mails, faxes and, for broadcasters, tantalizing chunks of ready-to-air film footage trumpeting the findings of the study: a link between fish consumption and a 50-percent reduction in sudden cardiac death. As anticipated, this effort had the desired effect. The story received prominent play on ABC and CNN, in Time, The Washington Post, The New York Times, Newsday and in foreign outlets from Ireland to Asia. The major wire services and radio networks ran pieces on it. Restaurant Business magazine reported a spike in restaurant fish sales, and gleeful fish marketers plotted to use the findings as rationale for a new publicity slogan: Seafood, Take It to Heart.
>
> But a closer look at the fish study reveals that it is of little real significance. The researchers looked not at a random cross section of Americans, but at 20,551 white male physicians, fully 90 percent of whom reported eating fish one or more times each week—10 years before the study was completed.
>
> No follow-up diet data were gathered because the study was not designed to look at diet per se, but at other factors thought to be related to sudden death. And there was a strong suspicion (mentioned casually in the study, and hardly at all in news-media accounts of it) that the relatively small number of doctors who didn't eat fish also had a less healthy life style than their more robust fish-eating colleagues. In other words, the report may represent nothing more than a statistical fluke.
>
> In a JAMA editorial accompanying the study, Daan Kromhout, a public-health researcher with the National Institute of Public Health and

the Environment in the Netherlands, did nothing to dispel these doubts. He pointed out that earlier investigations had found no association between sudden cardiac death and fish consumption, and that this study "does not provide clear-cut answers." Indeed, Kromhout's editorial mentioned earlier research suggesting that a high intake of fish may even result in a "detrimental health effect" due to, for example, mercury poisoning. Thanks largely to the journal's publicity machine, however, more than 50 million consumers failed to hear Kromhout's cautionary message.

Lundberg does not consider this a problem. "People are told that eating fish once a week is not a bad thing," he shrugged. "What harm could it do?"[3]

What harm can junk science do? Indeed! In addition to being deadly, robbing you of health care choices, creating a false sense of security, nibbling at your pocketbook, and robbing you of your peace of mind, as Lundberg learned, junk science can cost you your job.

In January 1999, then-president Clinton was about to be tried in the U.S. Senate. One accusation was that he lied in denying under oath that he "had sex" with Monica Lewinsky. Part of his defense was that oral sex didn't constitute "sex." About a week before the trial began, JunkScience.com learned that the January 20, 1999, issue of *JAMA* would contain a study titled "60 Percent of Those Surveyed Do Not Define Oral Sex as Having 'Had Sex.'" The study's media release stated:

> In a 1991 survey of college students, 60 percent of those asked indicated they would not say they "had sex" with someone if the most intimate behavior engaged in was oral-genital contact. . . .
>
> These data indicate that prior to the current public discourse, a majority of college students attending a major Midwestern state university, most of whom identified themselves as politically moderate to conservative, with more registered Republicans than Democrats, did not define oral sex as having "had sex."
>
> Almost 600 undergraduate college students were asked this question in an anonymous survey: "Would you say you 'had sex' with someone if the most intimate behavior you engaged in was. . .?" Many scenarios were paired with this question—anything from hand contact with genitals and oral contact with breasts or nipples, to oral-genital contact

to penile-anal intercourse. Nearly 100 percent of respondents considered penile-vaginal intercourse as having "had sex."

JunkScience.com was appalled and outraged—way beyond the usual distress brought on by the garden variety of junk science.

The supposedly prestigious *JAMA* was about to insert itself into the impeachment proceedings against the president on the subject of whether oral sex was "sex"—a social and political debate not remotely connected to the medical journal. Moreover, why would any self-respecting medical journal publish an eight-year-old survey of what 600 college students thought about sex? The college students didn't even all agree that penile-vaginal intercourse was "sex."[4]

JunkScience.com swung into action, breaking the news five days ahead of when the media were allowed to report the story. The only thing more surprising than the *JAMA* study was what happened next. The *Washington Times* picked up the story from JunkScience.com and investigated. The next day, January 15, 1999, the *Times*'s front-page headline was

AMA Releases Old Survey on Oral Sex Just in Time for President's Trial

Even before I picked up the newspaper that morning, the American Medical Association had already fired *JAMA* editor George Lundberg, stating,

> Dr. Lundberg, through his recent actions, has threatened the historic tradition and integrity of the Journal of the American Medical Association by inappropriately and inexcusably interjecting JAMA into a major political debate that has nothing to do with science or medicine. This is unacceptable.[5]

Thud! Flattened with a shoulder throw. The firing of Lundberg was undoubtedly a victory in the war against junk science. Lundberg had long used *JAMA* to advance his own business, social, and political agendas—disguising them as "science." Lundberg's dismissal was significant. Medical journal editors shuddered. They were not, after all, untouchable. Accountability existed for irresponsible publishing.

Some saber-rattling occurred in the medical journal community after Lundberg's dismissal. One *JAMA* board member resigned in protest. The *British Medical Journal* considered making an award in honor of Lundberg. Numerous journal editors fretted publicly over "editorial independence." But Lundberg stayed fired. Lundberg was reduced to becoming editor in chief of Medscape.com—a tremendous downsizing of ego, prestige, and, most important, the ability to promote a junk science–based agenda.

Yes, the junk scientists elsewhere still reign supreme. But you can fight them—and win. While the opportunity to pin a brilliant, public defeat on the junk science machine doesn't come along every day, there are other ways to fight. You only have to know how.

The most fundamental action is to defend yourself, your loved ones, and your business from being harmed by junk science—and that means being able to identify junk science when you see it or hear it. That's what this book is all about. Reach for it anytime you're confronted with news that begins, "A new scientific study says. . . ."

Once you've figured out what you're facing, you can decide whether to take evasive action, ignore the news, or attack. If you need help, you'll always find a ready, willing, and able gang at JunkScience.com.

I'd like to thank the many great people who have helped me over the years at JunkScience.com and those who helped put together this book, including Anne Fennell, Barry Hearn, Bill Holt, Steven Curry, Harvard Fong, Dan Fort, and Alan Caruba. A special thanks to Michael Gough, who has been a dear friend and great teacher.

Steven J. Milloy

INTRODUCTION

WHAT EXACTLY is junk science? In a word, fraud. In a sentence, it's faulty scientific data and analysis used to advance a special interest. Who cares? Maybe you should.

Junk Science Can Be Deadly

Two people died after they stopped taking blood pressure medication in response to alarmist reports of a scientific study linking calcium channel blockers with increased risk of heart attack.[6] The study was so flawed, the researchers were forced to apologize to their colleagues.[7]

A cholera epidemic in Latin America during the early 1990s—including 1 million cases and as many as 10,000 deaths—was exacerbated by the Peruvian government's decision to stop chlorinating drinking water supplies in response to the U.S. Environmental Protection Agency's labeling chlorine as cancer causing.[8] The Centers for Disease Control and Prevention says chlorinated drinking water is one of the greatest achievements in public health.[9] The EPA is now trying to restrict the use of chlorine to disinfect water in the United States.

Millions of people die and hundreds of millions of people suffer every year from malaria. Anti-pesticide activists advocate the banning of DDT, an insecticide that public health experts say is necessary to reduce this toll.[10]

Junk Science Can Harm Your Health and Reduce Your Health Care Choices

Some older women forgo the benefits of hormone replacement therapy for fear of breast cancer. Alarm was encouraged by pharmaceutical company Eli Lilly's effort to scare women away from HRT toward its new drug, Evista (raloxifene). (See Lesson 1.)

Phenolphthalein, formerly the ingredient of choice in over-the-counter laxatives, was forced from the market by the U.S. Food and Drug Administration because cancer-prone mice given unrealistically high doses of phenolphthalein had higher rates of cancer.

The popular morning sickness drug Bendectin was removed from the market in 1983 after lawsuits alleged it caused birth defects. But "Bendectin was the archetypical case of junk science scuttling a perfectly safe product," said Dr. Michael Greene, the director of maternal-fetal medicine at Massachusetts General Hospital in Boston.

Women were scared away from using intrauterine birth control devices by a 1981 study reporting IUDs greatly increased pelvic infection. A 1991 reanalysis of the 1981 study concluded that the original researchers, "showed an almost complete disregard for epidemiologic principles in its design, conduct, analysis and interpretation of results."[11]

The role of prostate specific antigen (PSA) as a routine screening test for prostate cancer is controversial.[12] Some say it enables early detection and cure. Others point to the lack of credible evidence that screening is associated with a decrease in mortality. Routine screening (with subsequent diagnosis and treatment for many men) is associated with considerable illness and death in the context of a disease that is often not fatal. The cheerleader-in-chief for the PSA test conducts research with funding from the test's manufacturer.[13]

A Tufts University professor crusades against consumer use of anti-bacterial soaps and lotions, alleging the products will lead to antibiotic-resistant bacteria. The professor has no credible evidence to support his claims and the media fail to disclose that he is also president of a business positioned to take advantage of his smear campaign against current anti-bacterial consumer products.

Junk Science Can Give a False Sense of Security about Your Health Habits

Encouraged by Kellogg's, many people think eating high-fiber cereals will reduce the risk of, or even prevent, colorectal cancer. These notions arose from highly publicized but unscientific observations of a British medical missionary to Africa. Recent studies report no reduction in colorectal cancer among those with high-fiber diets.[14]

"Florida grapefruit and 100% pure Florida grapefruit juice are certified as part of a heart-healthy diet," says the American Heart Association.[15] But this claim is unproven.[16] For tens of thousands of dollars per year, the American Heart Association allows its name to be used in advertising by Florida citrus growers.[17]

Pharmaceutical companies have long promoted the postmenopausal use of hormone replacement therapy to prevent heart disease. But the studies used to promote this idea are biased; they rely on women who are likely to have reduced rates of heart disease regardless of HRT use.[18]

Junk Science Can Hit Your Pocketbook

Organic foods cost an average of 57 percent more than conventional foods,[19] but organic foods are not safer than conventional foods. These higher costs could amount to $4,000 annually for a family of four.[20]

Ridding your home of radon gas can cost from $500 to $2,500, according to the EPA.[21] A 1998 National Academy of Sciences study estimated that since 1980 Americans had spent about $400 million on radon gas tests and on renovations to buildings where the gas can collect.[22] The study estimated that about 6 percent of American homes have radon concentrations that would merit corrective action. No credible scientific evidence indicates that radon in the home poses a health risk.

In August 1999, a Texas jury awarded $23 million to a former user of the fen-phen diet drug combination. The verdict cost shareholders—including individuals, mutual funds, and pension funds—of pharmaceuticals manufacturer American Home Products $8 billion in a single afternoon. In addition to the absence of persuasive evidence of harm caused by fen-phen, the plaintiff's physician testified that her heart problems predated her use of fen-phen.

Junk Science Can Rob You of Your Peace of Mind

"A woman concerned that her [silicone] breast implants were making her ill removed them herself with a razor blade because her insurance would not cover the operation."[23] But no scientific study links silicone breast implants with the illnesses the woman was concerned about.

After hearing on the news that chemically treated apples may cause cancer, a New York mother called the state police to intercept her child's school bus to confiscate an apple.[24] Even if it were true that the chemical used to treat the apple had cancer-causing potential —and there is no evidence it does—a human would have to drink 19,000 quarts of juice from Alar-treated apples every day for life. You still wouldn't have to worry about cancer because the fluid intake would kill you.

Worries over cell phones causing brain cancer spur some users to buy and use inconvenient ear pieces in hopes of reducing exposure to harmless levels of radio signals. Others fret about living near cell phone base stations. Still others wear metal-lined undergarments in hopes of reducing exposure to electric and magnetic fields.

To scare Americans into supporting a political agenda, former EPA administrator Carol Browner utters alarmist half-truths such as "Half a million children live within a mile of a toxic waste site in the United States"[25] and "We're very concerned about the one-quarter of Americans who live within four miles of a Superfund site."[26] But there is no evidence—none—that just living near a toxic waste site has harmed any child's health.

I could go on. There are many examples. But you get the point. You can't avoid the junk science assault. Your first question should be, "How can I avoid being hurt?" The answer is Junk Science Judo.

This book is a manual on the Junk Science Judo of self-defense. Junk Science Judo is E-Z. It doesn't require expertise in science. You don't have to know any statistics. There are only 12 lessons to learn, each with a few supplemental rules to remember. Earn your "black belt" and you'll be debunking junk science in no time.

How did I come up with Junk Science Judo? I learned the basics of epidemiology and biostatistics long ago as a graduate student at the Johns Hopkins University School of Public Health. I've studied the phenomenon of junk science daily since 1991.

I've observed just about every significant way science can be abused by health scare con artists. I've culled the most useful principles from these observations and presented them in the overall framework of KISS (keep it simple, stupid). The key to mastering Junk Science Judo is understanding (1) the basic process of science and (2) the modus operandi of the Junksters.

Science is the time-honored, systematic method of acquiring knowledge about our world. The process of science is simple; it doesn't require an Einstein-like intellect. Best of all, the process of science never changes. So you don't have to worry that what you learn today will be obsolete tomorrow.

Junksters typically try to sell you on the notion that some consumer product, everyday activity, or condition in the environment causes harm to your health. They try to establish cause-and-effect relationships, such as cell phones causing brain cancer, caffeine causing birth defects, or air pollution causing premature death. Junk Science Judo, therefore, deals mostly with causation issues.

The first step in trying to establish a cause-and-effect relationship is associating a product, activity, or condition with a health effect. This is usually done in one of two ways: (1) by testing the product, activity, or condition on laboratory animals or (2) by studying the health of human populations that are "exposed" to the product, activity, or condition. Such human study is called "epidemiology."

Animal studies and epidemiology may be valid ways of associating products, activities, and conditions with risk to health. But such associations are only the first step. They are preliminary.

- Laboratory animals may or may not be appropriate models for human beings. Mice aren't little people.
- Epidemiology studies produce only statistical associations. They do not provide biological explanations for the associations.

Much follow-up work typically needs to be done to determine whether preliminary associations are true cause-and-effect relationships. But that is exactly what the Junksters *don't* do. Jumping to conclusions about cause and effect from mere associations is the Junksters' MO.

Like any game, science has rules. Playing outside those rules is cheating. Catching cheaters is what Junk Science Judo is all about. Whether and how you punish the cheaters is up to you. But may I suggest Austin Powers' approach—"Judo-o-o . . . CHOP!"

LESSON 1:
KNOW THINE ENEMY

*Tricks and treachery are the practice of fools that
don't have brains enough to be honest.*

—Benjamin Franklin

JUNK SCIENCE USERS don't care about science. They don't care about your welfare. They're out for themselves, plain and simple. This might not be so bad if they admitted up front: "Hey, we're about to start a health scare. But don't worry. It's only a scam."

That's the rub, though. At their core, they simply aren't an honest lot. Deception is their stock in trade. They'll never admit they were wrong for fear the public will permanently turn a deaf ear to their "boy cries wolf" tactics. Instead they blame the public for health scares.

The Natural Resources Defense Council sponsored the 1989 health scare over apples treated with the chemical growth regulator Alar. When publicly rebuked for the health scare in August 2000, the NRDC responded, "The message of that report might have been muddled by the media, and the public might have over-reacted."[27] I imagine it's difficult for the public not to overreact when an ostensibly responsible major television news show features a congressman who links Alar with "bald, wasting-away kids" in children's hospitals.[28]

The basic deception among the junk science mob is motivation. They masquerade as newspersons "reporting 4 you"; concerned researchers striving to "protect" the public health; government "authorities" acting "for the people"; businesses dedicated to your health; and the "socially conscious," watching out for our children and planet.

Don't fall for it.

Since the scoundrels don't come with a scarlet "J" tattooed on their foreheads, you need to know whom to watch for. "Know thine enemy" is the first rule of warfare—and of Junk Science Judo. You can beat the Junksters, but you must know whom to engage.

Without further ado, let's meet the motley crew.

The Media: Ratings = Revenue

Many in the media fancy themselves public servants. It's a charming but naive notion. The media are businesses—and businesses have cares and concerns different from public services. As businesses, media outlets' ultimate responsibility is to the financial bottom line—not to you.

Broadcast media care about ratings. Print media care about circulation. Internet media care about hits. Ratings, circulation, and hits translate into advertising revenue and profits. If the media can get your attention, you can help their income statements and balance sheets.

Scaring you is one way to get your attention.

In May 1997, I was invited to talk about the media's role in health scares on *ABC World News Tonight*. Here's how it went:

> Voice-Over: World News Tonight with Peter Jennings continues. Now, "Solutions."
>
> Peter Jennings: We've been doing a reality check on "Solutions" this week, which means taking a second look to see if some "Solutions" turn out as advertised. . . .
>
> Tonight, we turn to all those health warnings which we very often pick up from the scientific community and put on the public agenda. The question is which ones to believe. We have borrowed John Stossel from ABC's *20/20* to give us his take on warning mania.

John Stossel, ABC News: Ever wonder if that cup of coffee is doing something bad to you? If you follow the news, you'd have plenty of reason to worry. It's been reported that coffee, or the caffeine in it, causes bone damage, miscarriages, heart disease, cancer and more. It's dramatic news, even though we don't yet know that any of it is true.

How can this be? Reporters weren't making this stuff up. It came from research done by serious scientists, often published in top medical journals. How could the conclusion just be wrong?

Steve Milloy: Because one study proves nothing.

John Stossel: Steve Milloy. . . points out that scientists get it wrong all the time. Studies have found that drinking milk increases lung cancer risk, that hot dogs are linked to cancer, that margarine causes heart problems. Sometimes it's because the studies are too small.

Steve Milloy: You can take any group of a couple hundred people, and you will find all sorts of crazy statistical associations. These studies are reporting statistics, not scientific truth.

John Stossel: Take the news about coffee causing cancer. Much of it came from a Harvard study that asked people who have pancreatic cancer what they usually ate and drank and then compared their answers to a control group's. The investigators then wrote in the *New England Journal of Medicine*, there was an "unexpected association of pancreatic cancer with coffee consumption." The media picked that up. . . . [Dan Rather, of CBS News, said coffee was a] "major cause of cancer of the pancreas." *Newsweek* said, "The findings can't be dismissed." *Time* quoted the study's author, Brian MacMahon, saying, "I myself have stopped drinking coffee." Scary. Still, no study is perfect. . . .

In the following years, a dozen other studies, including one by MacMahon himself, failed to confirm that coffee-cancer link. MacMahon now says he regrets titling his first article "Coffee and Cancer," but he blames the media for overplaying his research. Lots of people blame the media.

Steve Milloy: The gullible media pick up and go with it.

John Stossel: We're gullible?

Steve Milloy: More so than you know. Well, you need news. You sell—you're in the business of selling news and, frankly, it's news that coffee causes pancreatic cancer whether, in fact, it's true or not.

John Stossel: But we don't want to run with what's wrong.

Steve Milloy: It's news. You have to go with it. If you don't do it, someone else will.

John Stossel: Reporters do like to jump on the news. And shouldn't we be telling you what's published in a prestigious medical journal?

Still, we ought to point out that one study, or even five, doesn't necessarily prove anything. When there have been lots of studies, over years, and there's a consensus of scientists saying it's true, only then is it time to believe. John Stossel, ABC News, New York.

Peter Jennings: When we come back, the great North Atlantic monster.

Did Jennings listen to Stossel's report? Or was he concentrating on the "great North Atlantic monster"? You be the judge. Jennings started his evening news broadcast a few weeks later like this, "Good evening. We begin tonight with an urgent health warning about the largest-selling prescription diet drugs in America."[29] Jennings's report on the alleged link between the diet drug combination fen-phen and heart valve disease went spiraling downhill from there.[30]

Were there "lots of studies, over years, and a consensus of scientists saying it's true?" Not in the least. There wasn't even one scientific study. There was simply some preliminary and anecdotal information about alleged heart valve problems among 24 fen-phen users. The information didn't prove that fen-phen caused the heart valve problems. The researchers hadn't even compared fen-phen users with non-users to see if the occurrence of heart valve problems was significantly elevated among users. And what made the report "urgent"? Was it an urgent need for ratings?

Jennings reported the story because it was "news." His competition would report it; he had to as well. Jennings's employer, ABC News, is in the business of selling news. A health scare is news. It gets viewers' attention. Viewers bring ratings. Ratings bring advertisers. Advertisers bring money. Media moguls like money. The motive is not difficult to understand. It's the same motive that underlies popular television shows like *Seinfeld*.

The problem, though, is that while viewers know that *Seinfeld* is entertainment, most of them accept the news as the truth. No one thinks there really are four 30-something singles in Manhattan who, for example, knock down old ladies for a loaf of marble rye.

Most people don't think of the news as just another television show struggling for ratings. But that's what it has become. The line between news and entertainment was breached long ago. ABC's Jennings, NBC's Tom Brokaw, and CBS's Dan Rather vie for 30 million viewers every night.[31] It's big business. Sensational news is the standard fare. No genre of media—whether print, broadcast, or Internet—is above the fray. And there is a cost: Ask the many obese individuals who might have benefited from fen-phen were it not for the scare.

Millions of overweight people lost weight successfully with fen-phen. The media-hyped fen-phen hysteria resulted in one of the drugs in the combination being pulled from the market. Years after the scare, still no convincing scientific evidence proves fen-phen was a significant health threat. But it was great copy during the summer and early fall of 1997.

Only Scares Need Apply

The corollary of "the media love health scares" is "the media hate debunking health scares."

Dr. Michael Gough and I recently presented at a scientific conference the results of a study measuring the level of the much-dreaded dioxin in a serving of Ben & Jerry's brand ice cream.[32] Dioxin is the villain in a long-running health scare. A byproduct of some industrial and natural processes, dioxin is claimed by extreme environmentalists and the EPA to be one of the most toxic manmade chemicals.

Gough and I reported that a serving of the tested ice cream contained about 200 times more dioxin than the EPA indicated was "safe." The point of our test wasn't that Ben & Jerry's ice cream was dangerous, but rather that Ben & Jerry's was hypocritical in its claim in a marketing brochure that "the only safe level of dioxin exposure is no exposure at all."

I was interviewed about our study by seemingly interested staff of the television news magazine *Dateline NBC*. After about 20 minutes of questions, it finally dawned on the staff person, "So this isn't a scare? Then my producer won't be interested in doing the story."

Debunking doesn't sell. Worse, the media often do not even set the record straight when a health scare turns out to be bogus. Reporting a health scare means never having to say you're sorry.

Environmentalists Allege Cancer Risks Associated with Plastic IV Bags

headlined *Mealey's Litigation Report* on March 5, 1998. The scare mushroomed, producing more widely read headlines, such as "Vinyl IV Bags May Leach Liver-damaging Toxins"[33] and "Blood Bags Deemed Dangerous."[34] The alleged cancer risk was from a chemical called diethylhexyl phthalate (DEHP). A year after the initial headlines, a science panel from the World Health Organization's International Agency for Research on Cancer (IARC) downgraded its classification of DEHP from "possibly carcinogenic to humans" to "not classifiable as to carcinogenicity to humans."

IARC concluded that while larger doses of DEHP—much higher than humans would ever be exposed to through IV bags—were associated with increased liver tumors in rats and mice, the biological mechanism by which DEHP produced those tumors doesn't exist in humans. Absent other evidence of carcinogenicity—despite 40 years of certain human exposures—the IARC decided the rat and mouse data weren't relevant to humans.

The downgrading was unusual and certainly newsworthy in light of the earlier headlines. The only other time the IARC reclassified a chemical was in late 1998, when the artificial sweetener saccharin was similarly downgraded. You might even have expected that the major media— including the *Chicago Tribune*,[35] National Public Radio,[36] and CBS News,[37] to name a few—that so eagerly sounded the alarm earlier would reassure, or at least update, their audiences. But other than a lone report in an obscure trade publication, *Plastics Week*,[38] and a subsequent commentary in the *Chicago Sun-Times*[39]—by me—not a word of the IARC decision was communicated to the public.

The media exploit junk science–fueled health scares for sensational news—and then carefully maintain "credibility" by avoiding reports of the demise of the scares or their eventual debunking. The media are unique. They play a key role in virtually every health scare. The junk science mobsters need the media to hype their scares—and the media are only too eager to oblige.

William Randolph Hearst, the king of "yellow journalism," would be proud. "You furnish the pictures. I'll furnish the war," Hearst cabled Frederic Remington in Cuba in March 1898. It was a stunning display of irresponsible and inflammatory reporting that helped feed the U.S. public's appetite for the Spanish-American War. It's enough to make you wonder about the origins and wisdom of the war on drugs, the war on smoking, and even the war on cancer.

Advertising revenue isn't the only motivation for the media to propagate junk science. A reporter, an editor, or a producer may have a hidden social or political agenda that can be advanced by alarming the public.[40] A reporter covering a government agency may toe the agency's line and minimize criticism to maintain good relations with agency staff. Reporters may also be motivated by dreams of winning awards such as the Pulitzer Prize. Insidious motivation combined with uneducated and inexperienced reporters and editors, too little time, and too many easy-to-digest-and-regurgitate press and video releases from members of the junk science mob make the media the trumpet of junk science.

Personal Injury Lawyers: A No-Class Action

Personal injury lawyers use junk science to bamboozle juries into awarding huge monetary damages against deep-pocketed corporate defendants. Clever lawyers compound successful individual trials into class action lawsuits involving thousands of plaintiffs and staggering stakes. The threat of a class action award—which can lead to bankruptcy—is enough to cause some corporate defendants to settle a single class action lawsuit for billions of dollars, even where no liability exists. Plaintiffs' lawyers may net 30 to 40 percent of the total award. Not bad for what amounts to legalized extortion.

While the media generally leave their audience with the impression that settling is an admission of wrongdoing, that isn't the case at all. Publicly held corporations have a financial responsibility to their stockholders. It is often less expensive—financially and public relations-wise—to settle lawsuits than to fight them to an uncertain conclusion.

The now-classic case study is the saga of silicone breast implants. A woman received two silicone breast implants after a double mastectomy in 1978. One year later, the woman complained of a variety of health problems.[41] She sued the implants' manufacturer, Dow-Corning Corp., winning in November 1984 a $1.7 million jury verdict.

Encouraged by her success, others sued. By 1992 Dow Corning faced about 200 lawsuits. That year the number ballooned to about 10,000; then the U.S. Food and Drug Administration banned silicone breast implants. The FDA justified the action by saying the implants hadn't been proven safe by the manufacturers.[42] Emboldened by the ban, juries awarded plaintiffs as much as $25 million. Still no scientific data indicated that the implants caused the connective tissue diseases alleged in these lawsuits. As recounted by former *New England Journal of Medicine* editor Marcia Angell, trials hinged largely on "opinions without evidence."[43]

Plaintiffs' experts testified about novel theories, not data or analyses. In one trial, a physician testified that his patient began experiencing her connective tissue disease before she received her implants. The jury still awarded her $7.34 million.

The first large-scale study on whether silicone breast implants were linked to connective tissue disease was published in the *New England Journal of Medicine* in 1994. Mayo Clinic researchers studied 749 women with implants and reported, "We found no association between breast implants and the connective-tissue diseases and other disorders that were studied."[44] But the study came too late. The implant manufacturers were already on the way to agreeing to a multi-billion-dollar settlement of virtually all the claims concerning the implants. No subsequent studies have reported credible evidence of a cause-and-effect association between implants and connective tissue disease.[45]

With personal injury lawyers, science isn't important; class-action status is.

The Shallow End of the Jury Pool

Personal injury lawyers don't always restrict junk science to the courtroom. Junk science can be used to pollute the pool of prospective jurors. The respected British medical journal the *Lancet* published a study on silicone breast implants less than a month before a new breast implant trial was scheduled to start in New Orleans in March 1997. The timing of the publication may or may not have been coincidence—we'll never know. But the rest of this story is hardly innocent.

Researchers claimed a new blood test was developed for identifying exposure to silicone from silicone breast implants. The study was touted in a press release by Fenton Communications—a public relations firm whose clients include the Command Trust Network, a breast implant "support"-group-cum-recruiting-outfit for breast implant plaintiffs.

Fenton Communications' news release[46] proclaimed,

Lancet Publishes New Study Linking
Silicone Implants to Immune Problems

Two days later the *Times-Picayune*,[47] New Orleans' largest newspaper, dutifully ran a story with the headline,

Research Links Breast Implants to New Disease

But there were a few things that Fenton Communications—and then the *Times-Picayune*—got wrong. The study was limited in scope to the effectiveness of a new test to detect a specific antibody in the blood. It didn't link silicone breast implants with disease. The media release indicated that Fenton Communications was working on behalf of the *Lancet*. But one day after the *Times-Picayune* story, Fenton was forced to admit it actually was working on behalf of the Command Trust Network (i.e., the lawyers), not the *Lancet*.[48]

The initial press release relied on quotes from the study's lead researcher, Tulane University's Robert Garry. But it didn't mention that Garry was to testify as an expert witness for the plaintiffs in the upcoming trial against implant defendant Dow Chemical. Garry told the *Times-Picayune*: "We think this [research] backs up the claims of . . . these women that they're sick, that they're not making this up. . . . Our study suggests there is a new disease." But wasn't the study really about the new blood test?

Six months later, the *Times-Picayune* reported the jury's verdict with this headline,[49]

Jury: Dow Hid Implant Danger

Did the lawyers' shenanigans contaminate the News Orleans jury pool? We'll never know for sure. Certainly the lesson is that defense lawyers may need to bring chlorine to disinfect the jury pool during the selection process.

Activists: *Anything* for the Cause—and the Cash

Many people have causes these days. Some have turned their activism into organizations. They operate under benign banners like "physicians' committees," "public-interest" groups, "consumer rights" organizations, and even "mothers." Activists often place their agendas ahead of the facts. They will say and do virtually anything to promote their cause. If a health scare will help, then a health scare can be manufactured.

When scientific studies began to appear reporting no link between silicone breast implants and connective tissue disease, Sybil Niden

Goldrich, cofounder of the activist group Command Trust Network, told the PBS television show *Frontline*,[50] "The science? The devil with science. It doesn't matter anymore."

Then there is the anti-tobacco activist group, Americans for Nonsmokers Rights, that had the unwitting courtesy to acknowledge that politics is more important to its cause than science.[51] How did ANR come to make this confession?

Political Credibility über Alles

Boston University researcher Michael Siegel advised anti-tobacco activists on the ANR Web site: "Do not get into arguments with the industry about scientific evidence. . . . Instead, the best approach is to expose the tobacco industry ties of the so-called scientists making the arguments." In enumerating scientists allegedly on the payroll of the tobacco industry, Siegel wrote:

> Robert Levy and Rosalind Marimont released a report (issued by the Cato Institute) attacking the CDC and its estimate that smoking causes 400,000 deaths each year. All of these authors have strong connections to the tobacco industry. . . . Robert Levy works for the Cato Institute, which receives financial support from the tobacco industry and Rosalind Marimont is with the National Smokers Alliance which also receives tobacco industry financial support. (Note: Americans for Nonsmokers Rights can provide copies of tobacco industry documents which reveal the details of these authors' ties to the tobacco industry.)[52]

Levy challenged Siegel to back up his allegation. Siegel responded that he would correct any misstatements but didn't think he made any. Levy asked Siegel to provide copies of tobacco industry documents that allegedly revealed Levy's and Marimont's "ties to the tobacco industry." Knowing there could not possibly be any, Levy asked for a retraction.

Siegel admitted the article was misleading the way it was written and indicated that he asked ANR to post a retraction and apology. Levy accepted Siegel's retraction and apology, provided it was posted on the ANR Web site. Rosalind Marimont also took exception to

Siegel's article and he apologized. Was everyone happy? Not quite. ANR refused to post Siegel's retraction and apology stating:

> After further discussion [and] input from other [ANR] Board members, we have concluded that the possible "clarification" that you and I discussed is simply not feasible. . . . I realize that your views on the matter are heart-felt and sincere, and that mere removal of your name from the paper, without more, will not be entirely satisfactory to you. *But at this point ANR must put its political credibility ahead of what you consider to be your scientific credibility.* (Emphasis added)[53]

And there you have it, the activist attitude toward science in a nutshell.

"A" Is for Alarm

The classic case of an activist-promoted health scare involves Alar, a chemical used on apples from 1968 to 1989. Farmers used Alar to keep apples on the tree longer, enabling more efficient harvests. Apple retailers benefitted from the longer shelf-life of Alar-treated apples. Consumers benefitted from less-bruised, shinier, and redder apples.

Researchers reported in 1973 that laboratory mice treated with high doses of Alar had high rates of a rare blood vessel wall cancer. The EPA dismissed the results because the doses were ridiculously high. (You might want to jump ahead to "Lesson 8: Boycott Bioassays" if you're not familiar with how poisoning laboratory animals doesn't predict the future.)

By early 1983, though, the EPA changed its tune. The agency was reeling from a major scandal involving its toxic waste cleanup program. Looking to restore the agency's reputation, EPA staff recommended the very public banning of a chemical.[54] Alar was targeted. But the available data wouldn't allow the chemical to go quietly. Some EPA staff determined the alleged health effects from Alar were well within the range of safety. A panel of outside scientific advisers agreed with those EPA staff. They rejected the proposed ban. The agency withdrew the proposed ban in January 1986, only to have activists pick up the ball.

A campaign by anti-pesticide and "consumer" activist Ralph Nader forced many food processors to abandon the use of Alar-treated apples.[55] Nader described on the *Phil Donahue Show* how he personally threatened apple retailers:[56] "We're going to start a campaign to get Alar out of apples, but why don't you save us a lot of trouble and yourself by saying that you're not going to buy any apples or apple products with Alar from your growers." In 1989, the anti-pesticide Natural Resources Defense Council published a report titled "Intolerable Risks: Pesticides in Our Children's Food."[57] The report claimed, "Our nation's children are being harmed by the very fruits and vegetables we tell them will make them grow up healthy and strong." The report alleged that the cancer risk from Alar was 100 times greater than what the EPA estimated and that kids' exposures to pesticide residues would result in 6,000 "extra" cancers.

The report might have gone little noticed as just another effort to alarm the public about pesticides, except the NRDC hired the public relations firm Fenton Communications to push the report. Fenton Communications negotiated to give the television newsmagazine *60 Minutes* an exclusive on the Alar story. *60 Minutes* broadcast the report "A Is for Apple" on February 26, 1989, and the scare went into high gear. Frenzied media coverage and panic among the public followed. School districts pulled apples and applesauce from their menus. Apple prices plummeted. The manufacturers withdrew Alar from the market. All this based on doses of Alar given to mice that equated to a human consuming on the order of 19,000 quarts of apple juice per day for life.

Was the Alar scare about public health and safety? A memorandum from Fenton Communications about the scare revealed its real purpose. The memorandum stated in part: "A modest investment by the NRDC re-paid itself many-fold in tremendous and substantial revenue. The PR campaign was designed so that revenue would flow back to NRDC from the public."[58] Yes, activists need money to advance their agendas. Activist-initiated health scares have dual purposes: fear-mongering and fundraising. The former is the foundation of the latter.

Activists ironically criticize lobbyists as shills for corporations or other organizations. Let's get something straight. The only difference between activists and lobbyists is that lobbyists are better paid.

Businesses: Marketing Health Scares and Scams

The vast majority of businesses aren't part of the junk science mob. Usually, businesses are the victims of health scares. Products are unjustly attacked, typically by activists or personal injury lawyers. Sometimes, though, the attacker is a competitor. There are other business uses of junk science, too. A business may become so desperate when attacked with junk science that it resorts to using junk science to defend itself. Some businesses exploit genuine health concerns by making bogus product claims. Other businesses owe their very existence to health scares.

I grew up thinking only businessmen like Fred Sanford profited from junk. Boy, was I wrong.[59]

Cutthroat Competition: Hormone Replacement Terror

Women have used hormone replacement therapy (HRT) for more than 50 years to ease menopausal symptoms such as "hot flashes." Controversy exists, though, over whether HRT may increase the risk of breast cancer.

A recent review of the nearly 100 studies examining the cancer-causing potential of HRT estimated that among 1,000 women who used HRT for 10 years beginning at age 50, about 50 excess cancers might occur.[60] The researchers concluded, "The overall balance between the excess incidence of these cancers and other effects of HRT needs to be evaluated carefully and *will require more reliable data than exist at present*" (emphasis added). True enough.

The epidemiologic studies at issue almost invariably involve weak statistics, with results all over the map. Some studies report an increase in cancer rates among HRT users. Others don't. Still others report even a decrease in cancer rates. It's confusing. David Sturdee, the former chairman of the British Menopause Society, says: "A lot of nonsense is talked by those who say HRT is the best thing since sliced bread. Equally, I am incensed by the idea that all HRT is unsafe. Some women feel under undue pressure either to take HRT or not to."[61]

Pharmaceutical manufacturer Eli Lilly & Company is one of those applying pressure. The company hasn't necessarily been interested in "more reliable data." As pharmaceutical companies raced to take advantage of the HRT scare, the first drug brought to market was Eli Lilly's raloxifene, or Evista. Lilly touted raloxifene as having all the benefits of HRT with none of the risks.

Before raloxifene was approved by the U.S. Food and Drug Administration in the fall of 1997, Eli Lilly placed full-page advertisements in women's magazines playing directly to fear instead of facts. The fearmongering ads read, in part, "Many women have serious worries about a possible link between estrogen replacements and cancer." It's no wonder women worry; Eli Lilly's been scaring them.

Cutthroat Competition: Scaring the (Bleep!) out of You

The fiercely competitive pharmaceutical industry seems somewhat prone to fall into the junk science trap. This is because its products necessarily rely on scientific studies concerning safety and efficacy.

Researchers reported to the FDA in April 1997 that mice fed high doses of phenolphthalein—formerly the active ingredient in the popular laxative Ex-Lax—developed cancer.[62] The mice used in the tests were genetically engineered to be susceptible to cancer and the doses of phenolphthalein administered were many times higher than humans would absorb from prescribed doses of the over-the-counter medication.[63]

Despite the absence of human data indicating phenolphthalein-containing laxatives posed a cancer risk during more than 100 years of use, the FDA forced Ex-Lax products from the market. Correctol manufacturer Schering-Plough then launched a national newspaper advertisement campaign proclaiming:

A Government Panel has determined some laxatives cause cancer.

An FDA committee has concluded that phenolphthalein, the active ingredient found in many laxatives, may pose a risk of cancer. As a result, the government is considering regulatory action that may even include a recall of laxatives containing phenolphthalein. This would include most Ex-Lax products.

Fortunately, today there's Correctol Laxative which does not contain phenolphthalein.

Because of the importance of this issue, Correctol invites you to call 1-888-570-4200.[64]

Even the FDA was outraged at Schering-Plough's campaign to scare Ex-Lax users into switching to Correctol. Schering-Plough was compelled to pull the plug.[65]

Cutthroat Competition: Shoplifting Market Share

At least Schering-Plough didn't go to the trouble of creating its own junk science to attack a competitor—the way Checkpoint Systems, Inc., did.

Checkpoint Systems is the second-largest seller of electronic anti-shoplifting (EAS) systems.[66] The company gave up on competing the old-fashioned way—better products, lower prices—and commissioned its own junk science to scare the public about EAS systems sold by the largest vendor, Sensormatic Electronic Systems, Inc.

Study Says Electronics Can Wreak Havoc in Pacemakers

proclaimed the trade publication *Medical Industry Today* on May 27, 1997. A physician released a study reporting certain models of EAS, including Sensormatic's, disrupted the operation of cardiac pacemakers. "Checkpoint heralded the three-year study because none of its products came into question to disturb pacemaker operations, implanted in patients to help their hearts beat regularly," reported the article.

It's no wonder that Checkpoint "heralded" the study. The company paid the doctor $100,000 to "study" the pacemaker problem.[67]

The study was so successful at fomenting fear that the FDA went to the trouble of holding a hearing. Much to the chagrin of Checkpoint, though, the FDA—not an agency necessarily disposed to discourage health scares—concluded, "Interactions with EAS systems and metal detectors are unlikely to cause clinically significant symptoms in most patients." Checkmate, Checkpoint.

Cutthroat Competition: Reprocessing Fear

A study isn't necessary to attack a competitor if a business can muster sufficient political clout, as in the controversy over reprocessed medical devices.

An appeals court recently affirmed a $15 million jury award against medical equipment manufacturer Baxter Healthcare for defective "new" medical tubing that killed a patient. Oddly enough, Baxter belonged to a group of medical device manufacturers—including Tyco International, Johnson & Johnson, Boston Scientific, and Mallinckrodt—that used scare tactics to force restrictive regulation of reprocessed medical devices, including catheters, biopsy needles, and angioplasty balloons.

Reprocessors save hospitals money by refurbishing medical devices labeled "single use" by manufacturers. Each device is tested to ensure sterility and functionality before reuse. Device manufacturers lose sales when hospitals use reprocessed devices instead of buying costly new ones. Competition forces device manufacturers to hold down prices.

The coalition of device manufacturers successfully convinced Congress to get involved in the controversy. At a congressional hearing, a Johnson & Johnson executive testified, "I cannot understand why anyone would believe it is acceptable to clean and reuse a delicate complex medical device that was designed for use in a single patient and approved by FDA for only one use."[68] Despite widespread use, the executive could only vaguely describe a few problems allegedly linked to reprocessed devices. In contrast, a study published in the peer-reviewed *Journal of the American College of Cardiologists* concluded, "Restoration of disposable coronary angioplasty catheters using a highly controlled process appears to be safe and effective."[69]

But the sensationalist media facilitated the scare. A *USA Today* headline blared, "FDA exposes patients to risks of medical recycling"[70]—even while the newspaper reported the FDA "has been unable to find clear evidence of adverse patient outcomes associated with the reuse of a single use device from any source."[71] The device manufacturers—and some reprocessors, oddly enough—won. The device manufacturers and large reprocessors agreed to the FDA regulating the reprocessors just like the manufacturers, including premarket notification and approval, registration and listing, submission of adverse events reports, and other regulatory requirements.[72]

The losers? The smaller reprocessors who can't afford the expense and time associated with FDA regulation. Maybe they'll be "lucky" enough to be purchased by the larger reprocessors.

On the Street Where You Blame

Junk science can drive a business crazy—even to the point where the business defends itself with junk science.

Busy Streets Tied to Higher Cancer Risk in Kids

announced the *Denver Post* on March 1, 2000. "Children who live near busy streets are at significantly greater risk of developing cancer than those who don't, according to a Denver-area study, " reported the *Post*. Despite the *Post*'s report, the actual results were uncertain, including, but not limited to, the margin of error in the statistical association being larger than the association itself.[73] More important, the *Post* missed the larger theme of the study—shifting blame.

In the late 1970s, the electric power industry was besieged with allegations that electric power lines caused cancer, especially childhood leukemia. Evidence of the alleged link wasn't strong, consisting of weak statistical associations derived from data of poor quality. The public was frightened, nevertheless. Numerous multi-million-dollar lawsuits were filed against the industry. There was talk of forcing the industry to spend tens of billions of dollars burying power lines to reduce exposures to so-called electromagnetic fields (EMFs).

Costly government and private research efforts also were launched. The electric power industry's effort was led by the Electric Power Research Institute (EPRI), which brushed with junk science in the process. A 1994 study partially funded by EPRI reported that children who consumed more than 12 hot dogs per month had nine times the leukemia rate of children who didn't eat hot dogs.[74] The study easily qualified as junk science. But why might EPRI—not normally associated with such bad science—be interested in linking hot dogs with leukemia? Perhaps if hot dogs or something else, like traffic, could be blamed for leukemia in kids, then pressure might be relieved from power lines as a cause.

The good news for the electric power industry is that the National Academy of Sciences let power lines off the hook in 1997 by declaring the data linking power lines with cancer risk weren't convincing.[75] While the NAS essentially ended the panic over power lines, it apparently didn't end the effort to point the finger elsewhere.

Bogus Product Claims: Fiber Frenzy

Most of us are concerned about our health, and there is a health products and services industry in place to cater to our apprehension. Not all these products and services are legitimate. From "miracle" herbal and dietary supplements to "guaranteed" weight-loss regimens, we've all seen health product claims that are bogus.

Although these claims are often based on some sort of cooked data and analyses, they have a "snake oil" quality that makes them self-debunking for anyone who possesses the slightest bit of skepticism. More insidious claims, however, come with an official imprimatur, such as a government seal of approval. In the 1970s, British medical missionary Dr. Denis Burkitt promoted the idea that dietary fiber reduced colon cancer risk. Burkitt observed—casually, not in any scientific manner—that poor rural Africans had much less colon cancer than Westerners. He theorized that this was due to the Africans' fiber-rich diet. Larger, faster-moving stools reduced the colon's exposure to potentially cancer-causing bile acids.

The theory's intuitive appeal propelled it to become conventional wisdom. But research on Burkitt's hypothesis produced mixed results. Some studies seemed to support the theory; others didn't. None of the studies was particularly well designed—the studies tended to rely on study subjects' unverified reports of dietary and lifestyle habits. The NAS thought the theory so speculative that it declined in 1982 to make a specific recommendation about dietary fiber and colon cancer. Eventually, though, commercial interests pushed the theory and the scientific controversy became a memory.

In 1984, two years after the National Academy of Sciences decided against endorsing benefits from dietary fiber, cereal manufacturer Kellogg placed a message on its All Bran cereal claiming that scientific evidence linked a high-fiber diet with reduced colon cancer risk. The FDA took no action against Kellogg, though the action seemed to defy a longstanding FDA rule prohibiting health-related messages on food products. The NAS reversed itself in 1989 and came out in favor of a link between dietary fiber and reduced colon cancer risk—though the state of the science had not changed. A subsequent federal law allowed the FDA to permit health-claims labeling provided some scientific support existed.

In its 1997 effort to boost stagnant cereal product sales, Kellogg petitioned the FDA for permission to make the claim that some of its products contain ingredients that may help prevent certain cancers, especially colon cancer.[76] The FDA agreed in July 1999 to allow whole grain food manufacturers to make claims on their labels that "diets rich in whole grain foods and other plant foods and low in total fat, saturated fat and cholesterol may reduce the risk of heart disease and certain cancers." The FDA, however, didn't give Kellogg's petition the scrutiny that goes into the approval of a new drug. Instead, the agency relied on recommendations made by the NAS 10 years earlier.

The agency ignored a *New England Journal of Medicine* study published six months before the petition's approval that reported no evidence that whole grain foods reduced colon cancer risk. The study that followed almost 89,000 women for a period of 16 years was the largest study ever on dietary fiber and colon cancer.[77] Three subsequent studies failed to report reduced colon cancer rates among consumers of whole grain fiber.[78]

After Kellogg hyped a rodent study supposedly supporting the fiber–colon cancer claim, Dr. Elizabeth Whelan of the American Council on Science and Health pointed out:

> We in the scientific community agree that fiber-rich cereals can play an important and health-promoting role in our diets, but to claim that these cereals prevent colon cancer is stepping over the line. . . . We find Kellogg's reliance on a single, non-peer-reviewed rodent study to make such claims for a particular type of processed wheat bran to be irresponsible.[79]

Bogus Product Claims: Isn't Taste Enough?

You can understand why something as bland tasting as bran cereal might need a little junk science to boost its appeal, but what are the excuses for chocolate and grape juice?

Chocolates Could Be Heart-Healthy—Really!

headlined the *(Quincy, Mass.) Patriot Ledger* on March 26, 1999. The headline was prompted by a study presented at a national meeting of the American Chemical Society and conducted by scientists of Mars, Inc., a leading manufacturer of chocolate candy bars. The article continued:

> Scientists have raised that unlikely possibility with a series of studies reporting that chocolate contains the same natural phytochemicals, or plant chemicals, believed responsible for the beneficial health effects of

fruits, vegetables and red wine. The chemicals, termed flavenoids, seem to protect people from heart attacks, stroke, and perhaps even cancer and other diseases. "We have shown that some chocolates contain both a great diversity and relatively high amounts of certain flavenoids, and thus may confer cardiovascular benefits when included in the diet," Dr. Harold H. Schmitz reported Wednesday.

The research is unassailable on the narrow point that chocolate contains flavenoids. But it didn't examine whether consuming chocolate—or even flavenoids in fruits and vegetables—actually has a "heart-healthy" effect.

Some studies statistically associate diets high in flavenoids with reduced rates of heart disease. But it's not possible to credit the reduction in heart disease to flavenoids instead of some other "heart-healthy" activity or characteristic of the populations that eat high-flavenoid diets. It could be that populations that consume more fruits and vegetables also tend to be better off socioeconomically, exercise more, and to be more health conscious generally—all factors that would tend to reduce the risk of heart disease.

I love chocolate—because it tastes good, not because I think it's going to prevent a heart attack.

Dangerous Cardiovascular Effect of Second-Hand Smoke May Be Reduced by Drinking Purple Grape Juice

announced the Concord Grape Association. The media release continued:

A new, preliminary animal study suggests that purple grape juice may block a dangerous cardiovascular effect of second hand smoke. The research presented this morning at the annual meeting of the Federation of American Societies of Experimental Biology in Washington, DC (FASEB) reported that consuming purple grape juice neutralized the ability of tobacco smoke to increase the stickiness of blood platelets in laboratory animals exposed to second hand smoke. Increased platelet stickiness is a well-accepted contributor to atherosclerosis, heart attack and stroke.[80]

The impetus for this claim was the American Cancer Society's estimate that "53,000 people will die each year of exposure to secondhand smoke; roughly two thirds of those because of cardiovascular disease."[81] But as discussed later, a causal link between exposure to secondhand smoke and heart disease remains unproven. A potential "blocking" effect of purple grape juice is even more speculative.

The key to junk science–based health claims is that they are essentially unverifiable by consumers. They often can't be tested by scientists. How can you tell if eating cereal is the reason you never got colon cancer? You can't. It's a great scam. The claim is intuitive enough so that you buy into it, yet so unprovable that you'll never really know whether it worked.

Health Scare Parasites

Some businesses owe their existence to health scares. The food industry has successfully scared many consumers about pesticides, commercial fertilizers, biotechnology, subtherapeutic use of antibiotics in farm animals, and hormone-treated animals. These consumers are conned into paying higher prices[82] for so-called organic foods that have not been shown to be any safer or "healthier" than conventionally pro-duced foods.

Radon is a colorless and odorless radioactive gas naturally emitted from soils and rock. Radon can seep into basements through cracks and crevices in foundations. Since the mid-1980s, the EPA has scared homeowners about radon in homes causing lung cancer. EPA-certified businesses will come to your home and test for radon and recommend potentially costly mitigation steps. The EPA and these businesses have been successful in having radon-venting provisions placed in some local building codes. Radon testing can be an issue in real estate transactions. The tests cause worry and increase costs. Yet the human evidence that radon in the home causes cancer is unpersuasive.

Studies of radon in the home and lung cancer yield statistically weak and conflicting results. Risk estimates for radon in the home are based on extrapolating results from studies of uranium miners who are highly exposed for long periods of time to radon and many other substances in dusty mine environments. Recent laboratory research indicates this extrapolation may be inappropriate because of differences in biological impacts of high-level and low-level exposures to radon.[83]

Other "abatement" industries focus on lead and asbestos. While lead and asbestos may cause health effects under certain circumstances, the abatement industries have taken advantage of the public's fear of *any* exposure to lead and asbestos.

Politicians: Wag the Junk

Politicians are focused on getting elected. Whether liberal or conservative, this may mean exploiting health scares for political gain and pandering to or distracting the public. There's no better example than former president William Jefferson Clinton.

Citing a 1996 report allegedly linking Vietnam veterans' exposures to Agent Orange with various health effects, President Clinton announced veterans would be compensated.[84] But the alleged link is junk for many reasons, including a lack of correlation between troop deployment in areas sprayed with Agent Orange and soldiers' blood levels of dioxin—the contaminant of concern and potential indicator of exposure to Agent Orange. Health effects can't be attributed to exposures that didn't occur.

The *Washington Post* editorialized about President Clinton's announcement:

> The announcement came amid the flap over the president's lawyer's citation of the Soldier's and Sailor's Civil Relief Act in defending him against the sexual harassment lawsuit filed by former Arkansas state employee Paula Corbin Jones. News accounts made the connection, suggesting that the benefits ceremony with veterans present could help offset the criticism that the Soldier's and Sailor's act had been abused. Administration officials deny that was the thought, and who's to dispute them? But the fact that the decision [to compensate Vietnam veterans] was based on such weak grounds doesn't help their case.[85]

The *Post* again caught President Clinton committing junk science in the middle of the Monica Lewinsky scandal. A few days after President Clinton confessed on national television to an "inappropriate" relationship with Monica Lewinsky, the *Post* reported:

> While the first family remained cloistered on a Martha's Vineyard vacation, President Clinton's senior aides and informal political advisers yesterday weighed options for counteracting the intense backlash his Monday night address to the nation caused in Washington.
>
> Advisers described the discussions as in an early stage, and said no decision about whether Clinton should speak out further is due for several days or possibly weeks. More imminently, Clinton is still weighing whether to cut into his vacation next week for public appearances. *One idea would have him go to Woods Hole, Mass., on the mainland just across from the Vineyard, to talk about climate change.* (Emphasis added)[86]

Global warming, of course, is the theory that manmade emissions of so-called greenhouse gases are warming the planet and causing all sorts of havoc, including increased spreading of vector-borne infectious diseases such as malaria and dengue fever.

Government Regulators: Burgeoning Bureaucracy

Government regulators are a mixed lot. Their affinity for junk science varies by agency, by the program in the agency, and by the administration controlling the agency.

Regulators are inertially driven to expand their authority and budgets. Health risks are reasons to regulate or, at least, conduct more research. More research and regulation require more money and bring more power. The key U.S. government agencies to watch on the regulatory side are the EPA, FDA, Occupational Safety and Health Administration, Nuclear Regulatory Commission, and Department of Agriculture. Some agencies only conduct research, including the Centers for Disease Control and Prevention, the National Cancer Institute, the National Institute for Environmental Health Sciences, and the National Institute for Occupational Safety and Health.

There are times when agencies act responsibly and refuse to buy into junk science–fueled hysteria. This usually happens when the government's reputation is at stake. A good example is the controversy over fluoridated water.

Preventing a Fluoridated Fiasco

The U.S. Public Health Service advocated the fluoridation of water for decades.[87] Opponents alleged fluoridation increased the risk of cancer and other health problems. Some even claimed fluoridation was a Soviet conspiracy to poison Americans.[88] In 1993, the EPA considered revising the permitted levels of fluoride in drinking water. Though most studies didn't indicate fluoridated water was a cancer risk, one study reported increased cancer among rats exposed to fluoridated water.[89] The EPA nevertheless ignored the study and didn't regulate fluoridated drinking water as a carcinogen.

Certainly it's not unheard of for the EPA to use razor-thin evidence to classify a substance as possibly causing cancer. The EPA, for example, characterized the scientific evidence on the insecticide malathion as "suggestive" of carcinogenicity even though it only amounted to one more rat than expected getting cancer when fed unrealistically high doses of the chemical.[90]

In granting a "pass" to fluoridated drinking water, the EPA maintained the credibility of the federal government. What would the public think, after all, if the EPA were to say the Public Health Service pushed a cancer-causing substance on the American public for 50 years? In contrast, the federal government has little of its credibility invested in pesticides—even though the chemicals must be approved by the EPA. Pesticides are "politically incorrect" and action against them is good politics for regulators.

Versatile Statistics

Junk science isn't used just to cover the government's rear end. Like most individuals and organizations, regulatory agencies love to take credit for accomplishments. And flaky statistics are a good way to do just that.

Tougher Inspection of Food Is Bearing Fruit, CDC Says

headlined the *Washington Post* on March 17, 2000. The article continued:

> Two years after a federally mandated meat and poultry inspection system went into place, the number of Americans stricken by the most common forms of food-borne illness has declined by almost 20 percent, federal officials reported yesterday.
>
> The drop in 1999 was larger than the already considerable decline the year before, according to preliminary data collected by the national FoodNet surveillance system of the Centers for Disease Control and Prevention. Overall, 855,000 fewer Americans became ill from bacteria on their food in 1999 than two years before, CDC officials said.

The decline of 855,000 cases of food poisoning sounds like a lot. But did it really occur? Who knows? Certainly not the CDC.

Federal government officials have claimed since the 1980s that food poisoning kills about 9,000 and sickens another 81 million annually.[91] The 81 million figure is from a 1985 study by researchers W. E. Garthright, D. L. Archer, and J. E. Kvenberg. Three years later, Archer and Kvenberg increased their estimate by 22 percent to 99 million.[92] The CDC estimated in 1999 that food poisoning caused 76 million illnesses and 5,000 deaths each year.

So which estimates, if any, are correct? How can the CDC reasonably claim credit for an alleged 1 percent decline in cases of food poisoning when the agency can't know what the baseline toll is to start with? Doesn't that make it impossible to detect incremental changes?

As pointed out in a 1998 report from the National Academy of Sciences, estimates of deaths and illness from food poisoning are just guess-timates—not hard statistics from actual counting. But the estimates can serve dual purposes. The CDC either can take credit for reducing food poisoning or can cause alarm over an increase in food poisoning (and call for a larger budget) just through new guess-timates.

Medical Journals: Just Another Business

Some science and medical journals are confusing. They may call for good science, but then publish junk science. The *New England Journal of Medicine*, in particular, was convinced of the need for good science when it was attacked during the breast implant controversy.

Personal injury lawyers accused the *NEJM* of colluding with silicone breast implant manufacturers by publishing a study reporting no association between implants and disease.[93] *NEJM* editor Marcia Angell reacted by calling for more "scientific thinking."[94] Angell editorialized,

> Many people have become alienated from science and scientific habits of thought—at a time when we need science more than ever to help us find our way through an increasing number of serious and complicated questions involving risks to health and safety.

Dr. Angell needs to practice what she preaches.

A Journal's Cattle Call

The theory that bacterial resistance to antibiotics possibly results from subtherapeutic use of antibiotics in animals is an example of a "serious and complicated" controversy. Angell, nevertheless, permitted the *NEJM* to become "alienated from science." A study in the *NEJM* reported "evidence that antibiotic resistant strains of salmonella in the U.S. evolve primarily in livestock."[95] The researchers concluded, "The circulation of highly resistant strains in livestock constitutes a potential public health threat, especially to farmers, ranchers and animal handlers."

That widely reported study involved a 12-year-old farm boy who suffered salmonella poisoning. The salmonella strain identified was resistant to a number of antibiotics including ceftriaxone, the antibiotic of choice for invasive salmonella disease. Cattle from the boy's farm and three other local herds were tested for antibiotic resistant salmonella. The boy's salmonella strain reportedly matched the strain of salmonella from one of the tested herds. The researchers concluded the boy's infection was acquired from one of the herds. The *Washington Post* dutifully parroted the researchers' conclusion:

> Researchers have concluded that a Nebraska boy's infection by salmonella bacteria resistant to a widely used pediatric antibiotic came from cattle on his farm. The report heightened concerns of public health officials that the routine use of antibiotics by farmers to treat and promote the growth of livestock is reducing the ability of similar antibiotics to cure humans of infections.[96]

But the study's gaping holes preclude these conclusions.

The researchers couldn't determine how the boy became infected with the salmonella. There was no evidence he consumed contaminated meat or came into contact with contaminated animal feces. Although the salmonella strain isolated from the boy matched a strain in one herd, it was not the family's herd. The researchers reported the boy did not accompany his father on visits to the other herds during the two-week period before his illness. How the boy became infected with salmonella actually remained a mystery. The researchers couldn't rule out that "unknown environmental factors" were the source of the resistant salmonella. Cattle can acquire salmonella from birds or other wildlife. There wasn't any evidence the cattle were treated with ceftriaxone, the antibiotic in question, or any other antibiotics.

And despite the researchers' alarmism, ceftriaxone resistance among salmonella remains low according to the National Antimicrobial Resistance Monitoring System.[97] But none of this prevented the researchers from calling for restrictions on the use of antibiotics in livestock and pronouncing that such use was a public health problem.

The fault for exposing the public to this alarmism ultimately lies with the *NEJM*. The scientific deficiencies are glaring. Publication of the study, in fact, seems to have been more a matter of convenience than scientific merit. The study fit neatly into an issue containing three other studies on infectious disease and an editorial titled "Emerging Infections—Another Warning."[98]

In her call for better science, Angell cited as a warning Carl Sagan's comments on his darkest vision:

> It's a foreboding I have—maybe ill-placed—of an America in my children's generation or my grandchildren's generation . . . when clutching our horoscopes, our critical faculties in steep decline, unable to distinguish between what's true and what feels good, we slide almost without noticing, into superstition and darkness.[99]

So what's to prevent Sagan's vision from coming true if a preeminent medical journal fails to enforce the principles of sound science?

The Journals' Bottom Line

What is the driving force behind medical journals these days? Here's another excerpt from the *New York Times Magazine* article, "Hippocratic Wars":

> The truth is, neither NEJM nor JAMA (as the two journals are commonly referred to) can afford to be [boring]. Though no one's idea of a tabloid war, the competition between these two eminent medical journals for subscribers, advertising dollars and intellectual primacy is fierce. Typically, doctors have no more than three hours a week to read the latest journals, and there are nearly 4,000 of them competing for a physician's attention. Grabbing a chunk of that reading time requires careful wooing not only of doctors, but also of the rest of us. In a trend some critics consider troubling, journals are increasingly gearing their content toward general consumption, appealing directly to lay readers in a bid to increase their visibility and make themselves a "must-read" for doctors. . . .
>
> JAMA and in particular NEJM have long and illustrious histories of publishing landmark research. But while these sober studies often set the standards of care for the nation's practicing physicians, they hold little marquee value. What increasingly get the buzz are life-style reports— tantalizing and suggestive research on sex, food, exercise and health "breakthroughs," studies that tell us, in Dr. Angell's words, "what to do when we get out of bed in the morning." That these reports sometimes teeter on the edge of scientific credibility is easily lost in the fact that they have instant and obvious journalistic appeal.
>
> Clearly, there is a voracious public appetite for such news. A recent survey showed that Americans now rely more on the media than on their physicians for health information. The rise of managed care and

the shrinkage in time most doctors have available for patients have contributed to this trend, as has the legion of aging, health-obsessed boomers. And there has been an unmistakable attempt on the part of NEJM and in particular JAMA to cash in on this, by running a steady stream of reports and commentaries that appeal to the public at large— surprisingly mundane reports on the health benefits of walking, for example, or the dangers of making calls on a cell phone while driving a car.

Medical journals represent scholarship, of course, but they are also businesses, and most are beholden to drug makers for their economic viability. NEJM and JAMA had display advertising revenues last year of $19 million and $21.4 million respectively, the vast bulk of it from drug companies. While both journals claim a fire wall between their advertising and editorial departments, it is clear that the vast majority of drug-company-sponsored studies that get published are positive, not negative, and that NEJM and JAMA rely on the media to make these findings public. This in turn generates a steady revenue stream, both from advertising and from reprints of articles that drug makers buy in bulk and distribute to doctors worldwide. These funds support not only the journals, but also the lobbying organizations that back the journals, in this case the Massachusetts Medical Society and the American Medical Association.[100]

If this is what we can expect from our two most respected journals, what are the implications for the rest?

It's not that you can't trust science and medical journals at all— far from it. You just can't blindly trust them. A study is not more credible because it's published in the *New England Journal of Medicine* or *Journal of the American Medical Association*. Journal publication is largely a function of what an editor thinks will interest the journal's readers. Scientific merit may factor into the editor's calculations, but it's not determinant. Studies must be judged on their individual merits. Even those that have no merit at all are invariably presented as if they do, with graphs and footnotes and all the trappings we associate with scholarly pronouncements.

Scientists: Fame and Fortune

Progress in science is incremental. It takes a long time for real scientists to become famous. They rarely get rich. But a good health scare can vault an obscure scientist into the media limelight and into lucrative research grants, consulting contracts, and book deals. Just ask George Carlo, once a little-known Washington, D.C., consultant who continues to surf the gnarly 1993 scare over cell phones causing brain cancer.

A lawsuit was filed in late 1992 against a cell phone manufacturer on behalf of a cell phone user who had died of brain cancer. The lawsuit was spotlighted on the *Larry King Live* television show in January 1993. A media and political circus ensued.

At first, the cell phone industry announced it would spend $1 million to research potential health effects from cell phone use. As the media hyped the scare and Congress got involved, the industry raised the research ante to $25 million and hired Carlo to run the program. Not surprisingly, the original and copycat lawsuits were dismissed for lack of evidence. Yet the industry continued to finance Carlo's program.

But Carlo disappointed the industry. His research produced little of scientific value, especially compared with its funding level. The industry was not even sure exactly how Carlo spent all the money. Worse, his leadership of the program sparked criticism that the research program had been a public relations stunt all along.

The industry finally pulled the plug on the unproductive Carlo in 1999. Fortunately for the cell phone industry, two reassuring government reports on the safety of cell phones soon followed. A May 1999 report commissioned by the Canadian government concluded that no evidence existed that radio frequency (RF) fields posed a health risk under normal use.[101] The panel also found that cell phone transmission sites emitted RF fields of sufficiently low intensity that no biological or adverse health effects were anticipated. These conclusions were echoed in an April 2000 report by the UK's Independent Expert Group on Mobile Phones.[102]

Despite these reports, neither Carlo nor the cell phone scare has gone away. After the industry ended Carlo's program, he turned from cell phone researcher to cell phone hysteric. Carlo began raising questions about the safety of cell phones, promoting an unpublished study that, according to Carlo, prevented the industry from honestly claiming the technology safe. Joshua Muscat, the study's principal investigator, responded that Carlo distorted the study's results. "The results are essentially negative," said Muscat. He also called the idea that cancer risk is increased on the side of the head where the phone is held—a constant theme of Carlo's in media interviews—a "nonissue."

Even anti–cell phone activists don't think much of Carlo. Louis Slesin, the publisher of *Microwave News*, the leading newsletter spotlighting cell phone concerns, noted that just as the industry funding stopped, Carlo "started to say there might be something to cell phone worries after all. Pardon our cynicism, but we've wondered if the two might be connected."[103]

To Carlo's rescue came personal injury lawyer Peter Angelos, who had squeezed so much money from the asbestos and tobacco industries that he was able to buy the Baltimore Orioles baseball team. Angelos teamed with Carlo, hoping that Carlo's future "research" will provide the basis for class action lawsuits. Angelos said: "I believe the evidence is mounting that there appears to be some connection between mobile phones and health risks. We think there's a lot there."[104] He must be talking about the money, not the science.

Within weeks of Angelos becoming cocounsel in an $800 million lawsuit against the cell phone industry on behalf of a Baltimore physician with brain cancer, the *Journal of the American Medical Association* and *New England Journal of Medicine* simultaneously published studies reporting no association between cell phone use and increased risk of brain cancer.

The Mob Rules

What an unsavory bunch! The Italian poet Dante Alighieri (1265-1321) was so sickened by the junk science types of his era that, in the *Inferno* section of his famous the *Divine Comedy*, he placed the diviners, astrologers, magicians, sowers of scandal and discord, alchemists, and liars in the eighth and next-to-most-damned level of hell.

The only people worse than these junk science characters were traitors, according to Dante.

Junksters are many and varied. But how can you identify them? Are the "profiles in scourge" presented here sufficient? Should you assume the "expert" on television or in the newspaper who's trying to scare you or play on your fears is a scoundrel? No. Not in the beginning, at least.

"Know thine enemy" is the first lesson in Junk Science Judo because you should work to develop a feel for the junk science jungle. It's not a license for unfounded assumptions and ad hominem attack.

You must first identify a health scare's reliance on faulty data and analysis by using the techniques learned in your remaining Junk Science Judo lessons. Only when you can debunk the "science" behind a scare does the motivation of the scare's promoters become fair game.

As you accumulate debunking experiences, you'll develop expertise in identifying Junksters. Eventually, you'll be able to tune them out. Until then, study hard and practice, practice, practice.

LESSON 2:
SHOW ME THE SCIENCE!

*Skepticism: the mark and even the pose of the
educated mind.*

—John Dewey

YOU'VE LEARNED THAT Junksters can be taken down. You've acquired some skills to identify the enemy. Now it's time for the nitty-gritty.

The fundamental, time-honored process of developing scientific knowledge is called the *scientific method*. Learn it. Love it. Live it. Leave it, and you'll soon be heading lippity-clippity (as Brer Rabbitt would say) into the junk science briar patch. This is the basic lesson of Junk Science Judo. Master it and no fast-talking alarmist will blow a scare past you again.

Who died and left the scientific method in charge? Some pretty smart dudes whose ideas have withstood the test of time. Ancient and medieval scholars generally took the "predetermined conclusion" approach to learning. They arbitrarily determined "truths" from which more "truths" were derived. Astrologers, for example, believed as a matter of faith that they could predict the future on the basis of the movements of celestial bodies. Wrong. Today, the Junksters believe that statistics are science and that statistical correlations represent cause-and-effect relationships. Wrong again.

Advanced thinkers began to depart from this approach during the 16th century. On the basis of observations, not predetermined beliefs, Polish astronomer Nicholas Copernicus (1473-1543) figured out that the earth revolved around the sun instead of vice versa. Philippus Aureolus Paracelsus (1493-1541) rejected alchemy and pioneered medical chemistry. Andreas Vesalius (1514-64) rejected the anatomical dogma of the Roman gladiator physician Galen and helped establish modern medicine and biology. These are just a few of the giants who helped bring about the Scientific Revolution.

English philosopher Sir Francis Bacon (1561-1626) committed to writing some of what the new method of learning entailed. Bacon described an experimental approach that built knowledge from observations. He wrote in his famous 1620 work *Novum Organum*:

> There are and can be only two ways of searching into and discovering truth. The one [flees] from the senses and particulars to the most general axioms, and from these principles, the truth of which it takes for settled and immovable, proceeds to judgment and to the discovery of middle axioms. And this way is now in fashion. The other derives axioms from the senses and particulars, rising by a gradual and unbroken ascent, so that it arrives at the most general axioms last of all. This is the true way, but as yet untried.[105]

Bacon urged full investigations and rejected theories based on incomplete data. His experimental method eventually became the guts of the scientific method—today's step-by-step process for developing scientific knowledge centered on observations or data. Notice that the scientific method isn't rocket science. It's just the simple and common process of trial and error. A hypothesis should get the you-know-what tested out of it until it is credible enough to be labeled a "theory"— an elevated status in science indicating the best-known explanation of some phenomenon. A theory that is confirmed may be further elevated to the exalted status of fact or scientific "law."

The Scientific Method

Step 1.   Observe some phenomenon in the universe.

Step 2.   Develop a tentative explanation, or hypothesis, for the phenomenon.

Step 3.   Test the validity of the hypothesis—e.g., do an experiment or otherwise collect relevant data.

Step 4.   Refine the hypothesis on the basis of the results of the test.

Step 5.   Repeat Steps 3 and 4 until the hypothesis fits the phenomenon.

The state of mind necessary to implement the scientific method is aptly described in this excerpt from a recent *Los Angeles Times* article:

> [Physicist Victor Weisskopf] likes to talk about his old friend and mentor, Niels Bohr, the "father" of quantum mechanics—the theory behind the structure of the atom. Comparing Bohr to a prototypal present-day Nobel laureate, Weisskopf remarked that Bohr was a better scientist. The present-day physicist, he said, is brilliant. He has an answer for everything.
>
> But Bohr was the true genius, he said. "He had a question for everything."[106]

The scientific method's experimental approach is more about questions than answers. But that is where the junk science mob goes astray. They rush to the answers without addressing—or even really caring about—the questions. It's positively medieval. They might as well break out zodiac charts.

Caution!

"Wrong" science isn't junk science. The scientific method calls for trial and error until the truth is determined. More than likely this means many trials and many errors. Scientists learn from their errors. So "wrong" science is part of the scientific method. "Wrong" science becomes junk science only when it is used to further some special interest. Here are some rules for making the scientific method work for you.

Rule: *De Omnibus Dubitandum*

Doubt everything.

That's the wisdom of French mathematician René Descartes (1596-1650), the father of analytical geometry. Descartes developed four steps to problem solving in his esteemed *Discourse on Method*:

> The first was never to accept anything for true which I did not clearly know to be such; that is to say, carefully to avoid precipitancy and prejudice, and to comprise nothing more in my judgment than what was presented to my mind so clearly and distinctly as to exclude all ground of doubt.[107]

Doubting everything led Descartes to coin the most famous sentence in philosophy: "I think, therefore I am"—the only truth he could not doubt.

You will undoubtedly understand the importance of this rule by the time you master Junk Science Judo. In the meantime, there's one good reason to be skeptical of health scares precipitated by new studies—publication bias.

Publication bias is the tendency of science and medical journals to publish studies that report a risk ("positive" studies) rather than studies that report no risk ("negative" studies). Researchers recently reported, for example, that of more than 200 articles published in the *Journal of the American Medical Association* and the *New England Journal of Medicine*, 80 percent were positive studies.[108]

Publication bias has two causes. Researchers don't always publish their research; many factors may influence a decision to submit study results for publication. Second, journal editors and reviewers have their own reasons for deciding which studies to publish,[109] always bearing in mind that journals can't afford to be boring.[110]

Publication bias prioritizes fear over facts. Doubting is your first line of defense against health scare terrorism.

A related phenomenon is what I call citation bias: studies reporting a risk are more frequently cited or talked up by other scientists, because they are inherently interesting and, if true, may in fact prove important.

Recent rigorous reviews of salt restriction trials in normal subjects show extremely small reductions in blood pressure and even these reductions may be exaggerated.[111] Other less rigorous reviews include flawed studies and exaggerate reductions in blood pressure by 5- to 50-fold. A study of citations of these studies indicated the less rigorous studies are cited much more frequently than the rigorous reviews that reach less positive conclusions. The researchers concluded, "This appears to be the result of an attempt to create an impression of scientific consensus."[112] It's an impression calculated to deceive you.

Be skeptical of scary health news. Never give it the benefit of the doubt. In science, credibility is earned, not self-evident. Only a con artist would have you put doubt aside.

Remember: I think, therefore I doubt.

Rule: The Yoke's on Them

The burden of proof in courtrooms is always on the party trying to prove a point. A prosecutor must prove a defendant guilty beyond a reasonable doubt. A plaintiff must prove the defendant is liable by a preponderance of the evidence. Even a defendant who offers an "affirmative" defense—e.g., contributory negligence or assumption of risk—has the burden of proving the defense.

The burden of proof is no different under the scientific method. A scientist who advances a hypothesis carries the burden of proving it. You don't have to prove it wrong. Indeed, proving something isn't dangerous is akin to "proving the negative"—a logical impossibility.

Junk scientists don't like carrying the burden of proof because they typically can't prove anything. So they've developed a clever but faulty defense known as the precautionary principle. The precautionary principle says that when an activity is alleged to threaten human health or the environment, precautionary measures should be taken even though the allegations are not proven. "Better safe than sorry," the Junksters say.

So I could contend, for example, that secondhand radiation emanating from your cell phone might cause cancer or other health effects. Therefore, you should use your cell phone only if you are at least 10 feet from the nearest person—the "passive cell phone caller." I don't need any scientific proof. Just my bald-faced allegation suffices. (Remember: You read about this scare here first.)

Don't fall into the precautionary principle trap. A health scare isn't real just because you can't prove it isn't. "Better safe than sorry" is a tactic intended to get you to panic and act on a scare before it can be debunked. It's akin to a high-pressure sales tactic or an old-fashioned flim-flam. The con artist wants you to leap before you look.

Junksters have their goals and ruthlessly pursue them. That includes suckering you into the usually impossible task of disproving their scam. When faced with alarming "news" about a new health threat (especially one that might benefit some third party), keep the slow, steady, ho-hum scientific method in mind. Boring? Sure. Tedious? You betcha. Slow and deliberative? Be grateful.

Rule: Inquisition—Not

Inquisitors of the Spanish Inquisition knew all the answers. Heretics and unbelievers were stretched on the rack until they confessed their errors and accepted the truth. Under the doctrine of righteous persecution (long since rejected by most theologians), they tortured and stretched mortal bodies to save immortal souls. You might have thought that such attitudes were discarded, in science as well as in theology, long ago. Not so.

In 1989, almost 370 years after *Novum Organum*, the U.S. Environmental Protection Agency labeled secondhand smoke as cancer causing—three years before the agency completed its study of the subject. The agency reasoned that since smoking was associated with lung cancer, secondhand smoke must be too.

Having predetermined the study's conclusion, the EPA's anti-tobacco inquisitors spent the years from 1989 to 1992 torturing unco-operative statistics into crying out that secondhand smoke causes 3,000 lung cancer deaths annually.[113]

The EPA's torturing and stretching of the data did not escape the censure of a modern-day federal judge who vacated the EPA's conclusion, noting:

> EPA disregarded information and made findings on selective information; did not disseminate significant epidemiologic information; deviated from its [standard procedures]; failed to disclose important findings and rea-soning; and left significant questions without answers. EPA's conduct left substantial holes in the administrative records. While so doing, EPA produced limited evidence, then claimed the weight of the Agency's research evidence demonstrated [secondhand smoke] causes cancer.[114]

Unfortunately, the court ruling came more than five years after the EPA forced the data to confess. While the EPA's findings were litigated, the anti-tobacco industry aggressively marketed them. By the time the judge smoked the report, it didn't matter.

Like proper Grand Inquisitors, junk scientists know the right answers beforehand. They have their agendas, after all. The junk science method is often nothing more than an exercise in stretching and abusing data to make them confess. Unfortunately, there's no organization like Amnesty International to advocate "data rights."

How do you know when a conclusion has been predetermined? Sorry, there's no simple rule. Take comfort you've learned that prede-termined conclusions do occur.

To spot a predetermined conclusion, you'll likely need to do some background research. Get some idea of the state of the science. Identify the key players. Delve into the issue's history. Even if you can't find a smoking gun, you still might be able to deduce the crime, Sherlock Holmes–style.

Rule: Speculation Isn't Science

Beware of schemers who try to pass off hare-brained and half-baked ideas—i.e., speculation—as reasons to hit the panic button. I found myself with one of these con artists on a recent broadcast of CNN's *Talk Back Live* television program titled "Could Too Much Cleanliness Make People Sick?"[115]

> BOBBIE BATTISTA, HOST: Are you too clean? Do you keep your family germ-proof with anti-bacterial soaps, sprays and detergents?. . .
>
> Good afternoon, everyone, and welcome to *Talk Back Live*. You scrub, you wash, you disinfect your house and everyone in it. But your "oh, so clean" kitchen could be the perfect breeding ground for a mutant super bug. This is the picture painted by scientists alarmed by the growing use of anti-bacterial products. The AMA wants the Food and Drug Administration to take a hard look at whether anti-bacterial products are overkill.
>
> Joining us first today is Dr. Stuart Levy, director of the Center for Adaptation Genetics and Drug Resistance at Tufts University School of Medicine. He is the author of the book *The Antibiotic Paradox: How Miracle Drugs Are Destroying the Miracle. . . .*
>
> Let's—let's review here. What exactly are your concerns about these products?
>
> LEVY: Well, I think . . . anti-bacterial substances were designed and developed to protect the sick person in hospitals, and they've been used successfully. I don't see a role for them in the healthy household because in fact they aren't used in the way they should be used, for minutes of time, and instead they're being deposited on counters and places where they serve a wonderful purpose of selecting for the very bacteria which will resist them.
>
> So I think it's a change in the microbiology of the home that we don't need. A healthy household, in my opinion, can do well with soap and water, and the old, more classic forms of disinfectant.
>
> BATTISTA: So are you saying that these products, particularly when used excessively, will kill all the germs, including the good ones, and the ones that survive are going to be so strong that there won't be anything strong enough to take them out?

LEVY: That's exactly true. It's taking a mallet to hit a fly. . . . I think that what concerns me is where is the benefit and the risk, and to me the anti-bacterials will certainly clear away. . . all the bacteria: what we call the good and the ones that could potentially be harmful. . . .

Levy has alleged the scare. Now, Battista gets at the basis for the allegation.

BATTISTA: Why do we need good germs in our environment?

LEVY: There are studies now coming out of Europe—at least five, six countries—that correlate too hygienic a house with children that have much, much greater frequency of allergies, asthma, eczema, hay fever. And when they look at these children, they find that their immune system is different from other children. And from the more sophisticated knowledge we have now, it turns out that these children have not mounted, as we call, or trained their immune system in the way that other children have, like you and I, I think, in the sense that you have to meet certain bacteria as you're growing up, as an infant: the ones that have been around ever since we entered the bacterial world. After all, we're in their world; they're not in ours.

And so if we don't have that opportunity as a child and we meet them later, we're not going to respond in the same way. So I think that the more we change the microbiology, the kinds of bacteria we interact with in the home, the less chance we have of training our immune system in the correct way.

BATTISTA: So you're—but what you're basically talking about here is a theory right now. So would you go so far as to say that these products are dangerous, that we shouldn't use them at all?

Battista astutely picked up that the basis for Levy's alarmism is speculation.[116] He cited only new studies reporting statistical correlations—not scientific evidence, much less proof of cause-and-effect relationships. Levy continued to undermine his allegations.

LEVY: You see, when you use the word "dangerous," you absolutely should have the data, and I believe in that. I'm a scientist.

What we have are data which tell us that there is reason for great concern, and it begs for more and more science. . . .

Levy's conscience apparently got the best of him as he admitted that he needed "more science." And now for the coup de grâce:

BATTISTA: . . . Let me bring another voice into the conversation here, and we'll continue what you were saying. But Steve Milloy is with us. . .

You—you tend to think this is a lot of hooey for the most part, right?

MILLOY: Well, I think this is a lot of alarmist bunk. I think that there is no scientific evidence that shows that anti-microbials are causing any health impacts currently or in the future. I think the notion that we're killing off good bacteria and somehow that's causing a health problem—I have seen those reports, too—but those are very preliminary and really amount to just speculation.

So Levy, the supposed "expert" on bacterial resistance, was undone by an attentive television talk show host who discerned that he was only speculating, but advocating a scare anyway. How can you discern when speculation is the basis of a scare?

Speculation is exposed by weasel words that reveal uncertainty. A term like "correlation" requires that you have some idea of what a correlation is—i.e., an apparent statistical relationship between two phenomena that may or may not in fact be related. But other giveaway terms are the same words you use every day for wiggle room: "may," "might," "could," "if," "possibly," "perhaps," "potentially," and the like.

At best, weasel words indicate "informed" speculation; at worst, they mean the speaker doesn't know what she's talking about. When uttered by someone with a clear vested interest in promoting a health scare, weasel words always mean junk science.

Rule: Anecdotes Aren't Scientific Data

Health scare news reports often start with heart-wrenching anecdotes of personal tragedy.

Kids at Risk

was a *U.S. News and World Report* headline on June 19, 2000. The article bemoaned the plight of an Alabama family and blamed the neighbors.

For more than 40 years, the family shared the big house and two trailers a mile from the Monsanto chemical plant, on the west side of Anniston, Ala. In time, the 18 of them learned to put up with the rotten-cabbage odor that wafted through town. The plant, after all, is what stood between many residents and poverty. Besides, there were family troubles: Jeanette Champion, 44, is nearly blind and has what she calls a "thinking problem." Her 45-year-old brother, David Russell, can't read or write. Her 18-year-old daughter, Misty Pate, has suffered seizures and bouts of rage. Misty's 15-year-old cousin, Shane Russell, reads at a second-grade level.

The Monsanto plant has made industrial and pharmaceutical chemicals since the 1930s. But for decades it also saturated west Anniston with polychlorinated biphenyls. PCBs have long been linked to cancer. More recently, however, researchers have discovered evidence tying the compounds to lack of coordination, diminished IQ, and poor memory among children. So when the extent of the PCB contamination in Anniston finally became clear a few years ago, a hazy picture came into focus. Perhaps the multigenerational problems of some families were not the result of poverty or bad genes. Perhaps they were caused by the chemicals in the ground.[117]

Although the article goes on for another 24 paragraphs, you don't need to read any more. You've already gotten the two basic messages, courtesy of the anecdote: (1) chemicals cause "thinking problems," and (2) it's the chemical company's fault. For health scare purposes, what more do you really need to know?

Given the reporter's suggestion that chemicals cause "thinking problems" and everyone is exposed to chemicals, he probably decided that readers wouldn't be able to read the rest of the article anyway. So the salient points needed to be memorably dramatized right up front. Anecdotes work because they touch readers' emotions and include only selected facts—here, mentioning research that links PCBs with cancer and impaired intelligence in children.

Certainly PCBs have been "linked" with cancer—the same way Richard Jewell was "linked" with the bombing at the Atlanta Olympics. Both were accused and assumed guilty but subsequently vindicated. The scientist who first "linked" PCBs with cancer in 1975 unlinked them in 1999. It seems her initial study in rats[118] wasn't borne out by studies in humans.[119]

The article misleadingly implies that numerous "researchers" have found evidence linking PCBs with developmental problems. The "researchers" are, in fact, essentially a husband-and-wife team who have been on a two-decade crusade to link PCBs with developmental problems.

The purported "evidence" they've come up with is flaky statistical studies of children from poverty-stricken families who have slightly lower IQs but no overall intellectual impairment.[120] Given the children's low socioeconomic status, slightly poorer performance on IQ tests is not unexpected or unusual. It hardly constitutes scientific proof that low-level exposures to PCBs retard child development.

An anecdote is designed to appeal to your emotions and fears. It's a ruse to get you to put your brain in neutral and overlook the facts. A good anecdote generates sympathy for the "victims" and anger toward the "culprit"—often an "insensitive, greedy corporation."

Tainted Experts

Journalists may try to bolster anecdotes with authoritative-appearing quotes from "scientists." MSNBC.com's "Tainted Tampons?" reported in compelling fashion:

> Ruth B.'s periods had always been a nightmarish ordeal. The rural Wisconsin woman suffered from severe cramps and pelvic pain, eventually being diagnosed with endometriosis, a disabling menstrual-related condition that is a leading cause of infertility. "It feels like there's a hot poker inside you, jabbing you in the gut," Ruth says of the disease. . . .
>
> Instead of suffering in silence, though, Ruth—who asked that her full name be withheld for fear of reprisal by the chemicals industry— became an activist, seeking to help herself and her fellow sufferers. . . .
>
> But new studies have begun to link the disease—as well as a variety of other reproductive ailments—to environmental toxins, specifically dioxin . . . a by-product of many chemicals, manufacturing and incineration processes, . . . Researching endometriosis on the Internet, the Wisconsin woman read that one route of exposure to dioxin . . .

could be tampons and sanitary napkins—products she'd used for 15 years. Ruth says she launched her own Web page "to try to get the word out that dioxin is a problem."

The anecdote's life support system included

- Arnold Schecter, "a professor of environmental sciences at the University of Texas School of Public Health and a specialist on dioxin's health effects," who felt "studies were needed to analyze how much of the dioxin in [tampons] could be taken up by a woman's body."
- Peter deFur, "a physiologist and part-time researcher with the Center for Environmental Studies at Virginia Commonwealth University," who claimed the FDA underestimated the level of dioxin in tampons.
- Dr. Philip Tierno, a "researcher at New York University Medical Center who studied the absorbent chemical in tampons responsible for toxic shock syndrome," who was quoted as saying, "The vagina is a very absorbent place. No amount of [dioxin] is safe."

The "experts" seem to lend credibility to Ruth B.'s fears—until you discover that the three wise men may not be quite as objective or expert as implied by the article's descriptions of them.

Schecter worked with the Environmental Defense Fund, an environmental activist group that has long sounded alarms about dioxin.[121] DeFur is a former "scientist" with the Environmental Defense Fund.[122] Tierno is an infectious disease expert, not a dioxin expert.[123]

Certainly if "scientists" with links to tampon manufacturers were quoted in a story as downplaying risks, we would most likely look at their pronouncements with a heightened level of skepticism. A reporter would probably paint them as "tools" of industry. Here the "scientists" got a free pass because the reporter didn't fully disclose their affiliations.

Masquerading as Science

Anecdotes may be misrepresented as scientific studies. The 1997 health scare over the diet drug combination fen-phen was started by a *New England Journal of Medicine* report of heart valve disease among 24 women who used fen-phen.[124] The report was a collection of 24 anecdotes, not a scientific study.

Several doctors made only preliminary diagnoses. The physicians blamed fen-phen even though (1) there was no comparison of the incidence of heart valve disease among fen-phen users and nonusers, (2) most of the reported cases of heart valve disease weren't verified as actual heart valve disease, and (3) there was no clinical determination that fen-phen was the cause of any problems.

A key part of testing a hypothesis under the scientific method is collecting relevant data. Anecdotes aren't scientific data because they aren't collected under the planned and controlled circumstances of a scientific experiment. They're intended to persuade you emotionally, not intellectually—that's highly "junk scientific."

Rule: Assumptions Are Guesses

Researchers sometimes use assumptions to bridge gaps in scientific data and knowledge. Assumptions enable research and analysis that might otherwise be stymied. This isn't an unreasonable practice as long as assumptions are interim, stop-gap measures pending development of relevant data or testing for validity.

Epidemiologic Guessing Game

Epidemiologic studies involving dietary, occupational, and environmental exposures to substances often rely on assumptions. An epidemiologist researching a possible association between air pollution and death rates, for example, likely won't have data on how much air pollution subjects in various geographic areas inhaled. But data from regional outdoor air pollution monitors might be available. The epidemiologist might then assume that the study subjects were exposed to the levels of air pollution measured by the monitors.

Such an assumption may or may not be reasonable. This will depend on many factors, including monitor characteristics, subject location with respect to the monitors, local weather conditions, and amount of time subjects spend indoors versus outdoors.

The reasonableness of the assumptions will also depend on how the study results are presented and used. Alarming the public about air pollution on the basis of, say, marginal results derived from "guesstimated" exposures is probably inappropriate.

Epidemiologic studies may involve many other assumptions. Study subjects may complete questionnaires or be interviewed about their health and lifestyle habits. Often this "self-reported" information is not verified by the researchers. They assume it's true.

The U.S. Centers for Disease Control and Prevention reported in October 2000 that obesity rose 6 percent nationally between 1998 and 1999.[125] The CDC operatives telephoned 150,000 people at random and asked them how tall they were and how much they weighed. None of the responses was ever verified for accuracy. Not even a sample of the self-reports was validated.

The CDC admitted that "overweight participants in self-reported studies tend to underestimate their weight and all participants tend to overestimate their height." In other words, the data are inaccurate. The CDC researchers generously interpreted this error as indicating that the true rates of obesity are "likely underestimated." A less generous interpretation is that the rates of obesity, and especially changes in the obesity rates, are not well-known.

Use of assumptions isn't limited to data. A study's statistical analysis may also employ assumptions. This will be discussed later.

Assuming the Risk

Government regulators regularly rely on assumptions in setting health and safety standards. Let's say, for example, no study indicates that a particular chemical causes cancer in humans, but studies indicate high doses of the chemical increase cancer rates in laboratory mice. Let's further assume a government regulator wants to establish a permissible level of human exposure to the chemical. How could she do this on the basis of the available information? She couldn't without making certain assumptions.

The fundamentally necessary assumption is that, because the chemical causes cancer in laboratory mice, it must cause cancer in humans, too. More assumptions will be needed to extrapolate from the cancer rates seen at high doses in the animal experiments down to the much lower expected rates of actual human exposure levels.

These assumptions aren't scientific decisions; they are "conservative" policy decisions designed to err on the side of safety. The box gives a summary of the major so-called default assumptions used by regulatory agencies in assessing cancer risks from chemicals.[126]

Major Default Assumptions in Cancer Risk Assessment

1. A substance that causes cancer in laboratory animals causes cancer in humans.

2. When both benign and malignant tumors are observed in laboratory animals, the benign tumors are counted with the malignant tumors.

3. When data indicate a cancer risk exists, data that don't indicate a cancer risk are ignored.

4. Cancer effects observed at ultra-high doses are predictive of cancer risks at much lower doses.

5. Estimates of human cancer risk are based on tests of the laboratory animal species most sensitive to cancer.

6. Biological differences between humans and laboratory animals are ignored.

7. A substance that causes cancer by one route of exposure causes cancer by all routes of exposure.

8. There is no "safe" level of exposure to a cancer-causing substance.

9. The risk of health effects increases linearly with dose.

10. Estimates of exposure are assumed to be at the 95th percentile of exposure.

SOURCE: Regulatory Impact Analysis Project, "Choices in Risk Assessment: The Role of Science Policy in the Environmental Risk Assessment Process," 1994.

Multiple assumptions are usually used together. Setting a human exposure level to a chemical on the basis of a laboratory animal experiment could involve all 10 assumptions—it's quite a nonscientific leap of faith. The system of default assumptions arose in the 1970s in response to a flood of laws enacted to establish human exposure levels to potentially hazardous substances. In adopting the use of default assumptions in its risk assessment process, the U.S. Environmental Protection Agency stated that "in very few cases is it possible to prove that a substance will cause cancer in man, because in most instances the evidence is limited to animal studies."[127]

Despite the development over the last 25 years of much scientific knowledge casting doubt on the validity of these assumptions, they remain the heart and soul of government health and safety standards. The result is that regulatory health and safety standards are arbitrarily set much lower than may be scientifically justified so as to err on the side of caution.

Assumptions are just guesses and guessing isn't scientific. Real scientists work to evaluate and eliminate assumptions. They also prominently disclose any assumptions they use. Should their assumptions be disproved, it's no biggie. That's what science is all about, and they appreciate the advance in knowledge.

Junk scientists, in contrast, milk downplayed assumptions for all they are worth and move on. You're left holding the bag.

Rule: Hypothesis Searching Isn't Hypothesis Testing

The scientific method contemplates that scientists design experiments to shed light on a narrowly drawn hypothesis. But some researchers jump right into a pile of data without a specific hypothesis in mind. They hope serendipity will produce a hypothesis suitable for further research and testing.

Some of these researchers, though, skip the subsequent testing part and just jump to conclusions.

Hypothesis Hotdogging

A group of researchers wanted "to explore a variety of factors suspected of [causing childhood leukemia], including environmental chemicals, electric and magnetic fields, past medical history, parental smoking and drug use, and dietary intake of certain food items thought to contain carcinogens or protective agents."[128] They admitted the study was a fishing expedition. The researchers cast a wide net in hopes of identifying risk factors for childhood leukemia that would merit further research—a reasonable approach to developing a hypothesis for subsequent testing. No problem, so far.

They stumbled across a freak statistical association between hot dogs and childhood leukemia, reporting 9.5 times more leukemia among those children in the study who ate 12 or more hot dogs per month than among those children who ate no hot dogs. The researchers theorized the sodium nitrite used in processed meats could be the culprit. Sodium nitrite is metabolized during digestion into compounds that reportedly cause cancer in some laboratory animals.[129]

The study had many weaknesses—most significantly that it was designed to be only a fishing expedition and not to test whether hot dogs caused cancer. A glaring deficiency—even for hypothesis development—was the absence of significant associations between luncheon meats and childhood leukemia. A hot dog, after all, is just rolled up bologna.

But this didn't dampen the researchers' enthusiasm for their finding. They took their story to the media. "Hot Dogs Linked to Higher Risk of Cancers in Children" headlined the *Los Angeles Times* on June 3, 1994—just in time for the summer hot dog season. Hot dog sales took a beating.

How can you tell when a hypothesis search has been inappropriately used?

Expect the Unexpected

Study results described as "unexpected" should be considered hypotheses to be tested. If results are unexpected, that probably means the study wasn't designed with those results in mind. If a study isn't designed to test an idea, it probably can't. If a study with "unexpected" results makes the news—especially if it hasn't been checked and rechecked by other researchers—you're probably witnessing junk science.

Statistics Aren't Science

No study that reports only statistical results can prove a cause-and-effect relationship. Statistical results are usually preliminary in nature and need further testing before conclusions about cause-and-effect relationships can be drawn. Preliminary results equate to hypothesis, not scientific fact. (Much more on this later!)

Data Mining

Another clue is the use of large data sets, such as the so-called Nurses Health Study and the Cancer Prevention Study II. The Nurses Health Study contains health and lifestyle data initially collected in 1976 from about 90,000 nurses and periodically updated through questionnaires returned to Harvard University researchers. The Cancer Prevention Study II was constructed by the American Cancer Society, which had 70,000 volunteers interview 2 million friends and family about their health and lifestyle characteristics.

There are several problems with data sets like these:

- The data collected are rarely, if ever, verified for accuracy. Every two years or so, the women who participate in the Nurses Health Study are asked to report, for example, how much alcohol they consume. But no one attempts to verify the responses. The data in the Cancer Prevention Study II weren't collected in a uniform manner by trained data collection technicians.
- These data sets were not specifically designed for the myriad hypotheses that are tested with their data. Often, the data must

be jimmied or interpolated before they can be used. Using the Nurses Health Study, for example, researchers reported that vitamin E, but not vitamin A and vitamin C, was associated with a reduced risk of heart disease.[130] The problem, though, is the researchers had no idea of the women's vitamin intakes, which could only be assumed on the basis of responses to questions on the types of food the women recalled they ate.

- The subjects that make up these data sets aren't necessarily representative of the population at large. The Nurses Health Study includes only nurses. The Physicians' Health Study includes only physicians. The Adventist Health Study includes only Seventh Day Adventists. See the pattern? Physicians and nurses tend to be more aware of health matters. Seventh Day Adventists don't drink, eat meat, or smoke. These data have built-in biases that affect study results.

- Large data sets lend themselves to so-called data dredging or data mining—that is, unbridled inspection of a data set in hopes of identifying some sort of notable statistical association. Thanks to improvements in computing power, data sets can be analyzed endlessly until something interesting pops up. Data dredging may be a useful practice if intended for hypothesis generation; it becomes a junk science no-no when, as in the hot dog example, it is converted into headlines.

Researchers shouldn't reach conclusions from hypothesis searching. It's like judging a book by its cover.

Rule: Use Yardsticks, Not Divining Rods

Science is an objective, not a subjective, process. It is about observing the observable and measuring the measurable in universal ways that aren't unique to the beholder. Counting the number of angels that can dance on the head of a pin, for example, is not a scientific process. Since you can't observe angels, you must *believe* they exist. Not everyone does. Belief is a subjective, not an objective, process.

So-called multiple chemical sensitivity is a classic example of unacceptable subjectivity in action. MCS is a modern phenomenon; scents, usually perfumes or other chemical odors, allegedly cause allergy, asthma, and other health conditions.

The claimed illnesses are usually diagnosed by individuals themselves or with the assistance of so-called clinical ecologists—i.e., shareholders in the MCS industry. But no generally accepted test of physiological function can be shown to correlate with the wide variety of symptoms presented by the patients. The only objective thing that can be said about MCS is that it has yet to be generally accepted as a medical condition.

How can you tell whether a health scare is subjective in nature? If it lacks any one of the following three characteristics, it probably is.

Health Effects Must Be Capable of Observation

Dangerous Baby Bottles? Scientists Try to Determine If Clear Plastics Can Do Harm

blared the *Patriot Ledger* on August 17, 1999. The article continued:

> They're light enough for a baby to hold and won't break if you drop them. They're cheap and popular, and some come decorated with cute pictures of Teletubbies and Disney characters. But recent studies have shown that clear, plastic baby bottles made of polycarbonate are leaching small amounts of a chemical into formula when they are warmed. The chemical, bisphenol-A, mimics the female hormone estrogen. *Some say it could* adversely affect a baby's development.
>
> *While it's still too early to tell* how dangerous the chemical can be to infants, consumer groups are calling for manufacturers to stop using polycarbonate plastic and advising parents to use other types of bottles. . . . "Baby bottles shouldn't release any chemical in any amount," said Jeff Wise, policy director of the National Environmental Trust. . . . "A young baby's body is rapidly developing in response to tiny, perfectly timed hormonal signals. We have no way to know *the subtle ways* that an artificial hormone-like substance, like bisphenol-A, can interfere with that development." (Emphasis added)

Not only have no health effects been observed, none are likely to be observed in the future. This probability is exposed by the use of the term "subtle"—the red flag for unobservable health effects and junk science. "Subtle" is another way of saying, "We can't observe any health effects, but we want you to believe they exist anyway."

Health Effects Must Be Capable of Measurement

Study Links Deaths to Airborne Particles

screamed the *Los Angeles Times* on December 14, 2000. The article went on, "Dust and soot in the air contribute to between 20 and 200 early deaths each day in America's biggest cities, according to the largest coast-to-coast scientific study of the problem." But measuring the number of deaths attributable to normal levels of air pollution isn't possible—and not only because the Grim Reaper doesn't stamp "Air Pollution" on corpses.

The researchers compared death rates from heart and lung diseases with air pollution levels measured by regional monitors for the 20 largest counties in the United States. The researchers reported an approximate 1 percent difference in death rates between the counties with the highest and the lowest levels of air pollution.[131]

This alleged difference is too small to measure by the technique employed. For this type of research study—i.e., epidemiology—increases on the order of 100 percent and less are considered too small to measure. Such increases may be due to chance, statistical bias, or effects of confounding factors that are sometimes not evident. So epidemiologic differences on the order of 1 percent aren't results; they're random error.

Because the researchers didn't reliably measure genuine differences in death rates due to air pollution among the counties, they couldn't estimate how many deaths air pollution "contributed" to, if any.

Health Effects Shouldn't Involve Interpretation

The problem of relying on interpretation is aptly described in a *New York Times* article from January 2, 2001,

Researcher Challenges a Host of Psychological Studies

The article reads in part:

> Here is the problem, as Dr. Linda Bartoshuk sees it: Say that two men, call them Richard and John, are both suffering from depression, and a researcher wants to find out if a particular medication will offer them relief.
>
> Asked to rate the intensity of his depression on a scale of 1 to 10, Richard selects a 6. John, given the same rating scale, also picks a 6. But does he feel the same degree of depression as John? Many researchers, said Dr. Bartoshuk, a psychologist at the Yale University School of Medicine and an expert on taste perception, assume the answer is yes, that, in effect, a 6 is a 6 is a 6.
>
> But in fact, Dr. Bartoshuk said, nobody really knows, since depression, like many internal experiences, is subjective.

Arbitrarily assigning numerical ratings or other like interpretations to health conditions isn't objective because they vary between study subjects and researchers. There's no common scale and no way to reconcile different interpretations.

Researchers may claim that such subjectivity is unavoidable. Perhaps that's true. But desperation doesn't give them license to call it science.

Rule: Study Results Must Be Replicated

One study means nothing. Science is not a quick-and-dirty endeavor. It's a process of incremental progress whereby study results are checked and rechecked to make sure that bogus conclusions do not make it up the food chain of scientific knowledge.

Study results must be replicated. At a minimum this means that subsequent researchers using the same data and methods should get about the same results as the original researchers. And even subsequent testing of the original hypothesis using different data or methods, or both, should produce the same—or at least consistent—results.

The Law the Junk Left Behind

The requirement of replication automatically precludes any one study from being prematurely enshrined as "science." Here's what can happen when this rule is violated.

Environmental Estrogens May Pose Greater Risk, Study Shows

headlined the *Washington Post* on June 7, 1996. Tulane University researchers reported in the prominent journal *Science* seemingly alarming results about so-called endocrine disrupters or environmental estrogens—manmade chemicals, like pesticides, PCBs, and plasticizers that allegedly disrupt hormonal systems to cause everything from cancer to infertility to attention deficit disorder.[132]

On the basis of their laboratory experiment, the Tulane researchers claimed that mixtures of manmade chemicals—specifically PCBs and pesticides—were 1,000 times more potent as hormone disrupters than any of the chemicals alone. This news was alarming because humans are exposed to many different chemicals in the environment every day.

While most *Science* studies are published without additional editorial and news coverage, *Science* announced the study with a great deal of fanfare, also publishing a related news story and commentary. The study attracted the attention of government regulators.

"The new study is the strongest evidence to date that combinations of estrogenic chemicals may be potent enough to significantly increase the risk of breast cancer, prostate cancer, birth defects and other major health concerns," said then–U.S. Environmental Protection Agency administrator Carol M. Browner.[133]

"I was astounded by the findings," said Dr. Lynn Goldman, then the EPA's pesticide chief. "I just can't remember a time where I've seen data so persuasive as far as making an argument for synergy between chemicals. The results are very clean-looking."[134]

The story was widely published and created a stir. Even lawmakers responded. In the wake of the publicity, the Food Quality Protection Act of 1996 was enacted, requiring the EPA to develop programs for screening chemicals for estrogenic activity. The law was enacted before anyone could raise questions about the study.

Eventually, though, the study began to unravel.

In January 1997, scientists from four independent laboratories officially reported the study's results couldn't be replicated.[135] Two weeks later, British researchers reported in the journal *Nature* that they could not replicate the Tulane researchers' findings.[136] Finally, in July 1997, the Tulane researchers were compelled to retract their study, writing in *Science*, "We . . . have not been able to replicate our initial results . . . [and] others have been unable to reproduce the results we reported."[137] "I really can't explain the original findings," the lead researcher said in an interview.[138]

We'll probably never know whether the study resulted from mistakes or fraud. In any case, the scientific community rejected the study. But in contrast to the media coverage of the study, no one ballyhooed the rebuttal and retraction. The *Washington Post*, so eager to cover the original findings, didn't report the retraction for three weeks.[139]

While the study is gone, the law and the EPA regulatory program remain.

Wanted: Contraception for Junk Science

The need for studies to be replicated is so important that I'll emphasize the point with another example.

The Dalkon Shield was an intrauterine birth control device (IUD) marketed by the A.H. Robins Company beginning in 1971. The product was withdrawn from the market in 1974 because of anecdotal reports of health problems among users.

In 1976, the National Institutes of Health commenced the Women's Health Study to investigate a possible association between IUDs and pelvic infections. The study, published in 1981, reported that

IUDs, in general, increased the risk of pelvic infections by 60 percent.[140] The study played a central role in litigation that forced A.H. Robins into bankruptcy.[141]

In 1991 researchers reexamined the original data from the Women's Health Study and found that some women had been eliminated from the study without any scientific basis. The researchers who reexamined the data also suggested that adverse publicity about IUDs at the time of the Women's Health Study could have biased patients' recall about their medical history and biased doctors to diagnose infections in women who used the Dalkon Shield. Summing up the reexamination, the authors of the 1991 report in the *Journal of Clinical Epidemiology* said that the Women's Health Study "showed almost a complete disregard for epidemiological principles in its design, conduct, analysis and interpretation of results."[142]

But the reanalysis was years too late. In 1989 A.H. Robins was purchased by American Home Products in what was termed a "steal deal."[143] The Dalkon Shield, an effective birth control device, was never reintroduced to the market.

Rule: Replication Must Be Independent

It's not enough that studies are replicated. The replication must be conducted by researchers who are independent from the original researchers. This prevents bias from creeping into the replication process. Nonindependent replication is sort of like students grading their own exams at home.

"Independent" means *genuinely* disinterested in the outcome of the replication. Genuine disinterest is a tough criterion to judge. Practically speaking, I like to see that the subsequent researchers have no significant affiliation with the original researchers. At a minimum this means the researchers should be from different institutions and have different funding sources.

See how much confidence you have in the replication efforts behind the science underlying the FDA's recent effort to require that foods be labeled as to their content of trans fatty acids or "trans fats" —vegetable fats treated to keep pastries firm and margarine stiff at room temperature.

An editorial published in the *New England Journal of Medicine* before the FDA proposed the new labeling rule reviewed six epidemiologic studies on trans fats and heart disease. Its authors concluded that "epidemiologic studies indicate an adverse effect of trans fatty acids on the risk of coronary heart disease."[144] Table 2.1 summarizes the results of the six studies.

Check out the authors of the studies listed in the table. See if you notice anything unusual (Hint: compare the names in bold with the study outcome). All the epidemiologic studies reporting a link between trans fats and heart disease risk are authored by Alberto Ascherio and Walter Willett. You might also be interested in knowing who authored the *New England Journal of Medicine* editorial: Alberto Ascherio, Martijn B. Katan, Peter L. Zock, Meir J. Stampfer, and Walter C. Willett.

Is this science or the Ascherio-Willett railroad? Are the conductors right? Who knows? One thing's for sure, though. A better system of comment on scientific research than self-review can be found.

No Madness in the Scientific Method

The scientific method places the burden of proving the truth of a scientific theory on its advocates—not on you. Your job is to doubt until they've met the burden of proof. Theories, anecdotes, and assumptions aren't proof of anything. The scientific method requires that scientists develop narrowly drawn hypotheses to be tested by appropriately designed and conducted experiments and analyses. The results must then be reviewed and replicated by others. Then the process starts all over—with everyone incrementally smarter, we hope.

When does it end? When the hypothesis perfectly explains the results. Until then, the yoke's on them. When faced with speculation or hypotheses masquerading as fact, you owe it to yourself to make one clear demand: Show me the science!

Table 2.1: Epidemiologic Studies on Trans Fats and Heart Disease

Study	Authors Conclude a Link
Ascherio, A., C. H. Hennekens, J. E. Buring, C. Master, M. J. Stampfer, **W. C. Willett**. "Trans-fatty Acids Intake and Risk of Myocardial Infarction." *Circulation* 89 (1994): 94–101.	Yes
Bolton-Smith, C., M. Woodward, S. Fenton, C. A. Brown. "Does Dietary Trans Fatty Acid Intake Relate to the Prevalence of Coronary Heart Disease in Scotland?" *European Heart Journal* 17 (1996): 837–45.	No
Aro, A., A. F. Kardinaal, I. Salminen, et al. "Adipose Tissue Isomeric Trans Fatty Acids and Risk of Myocardial Infarction in Nine Countries: The EURAMIC Study." *Lancet* 345 (1995): 273–78.	No
Ascherio, A., E. B. Rimm, E. L. Giovannucci, D. Spiegelman, M. Stampfer, **W. C. Willett**. "Dietary Fat and Risk of Coronary Heart Disease in Men: Cohort Follow Up Study in the United States." *British Medical Journal* 313 (1996): 84–89	Yes
Pietinen, P., **A. Ascherio**, P. Korhonen, A. M. Hartman, **W. C. Willett**, D. Albanes, J. Virtamo. "Intake of Fatty Acids and Risk of Coronary Heart Disease in a Cohort of Finnish Men: The Alpha-Tocopherol, Beta-Carotene Cancer Prevention Study." *American Journal of Epidemiology* 145 (1997): 876–87.	Yes
Hu, F. B., M. J. Stampfer, J. E. Manson, E. Rimm, G. A. Colditz, B. A. Rosner, C. H. Hennekens, **W. C. Willett**. "Dietary Fat Intake and the Risk of Coronary Heart Disease in Women." *New England Journal of Medicine* 337 (1997): 1491–99.	Yes

LESSON 3:
STATISTICS AREN'T SCIENCE

Statistics are like bikinis. What they reveal is
suggestive, but what they conceal is vital.

—Aaron Levenstein

STATISTICS ARE THE lingua franca of junk science. They make good sound bites, adding a quantitative feel to otherwise "fuzzy" health scares. Credibility is added ostensibly by a statistic's neutral nature and authoritative source. The result is an inappropriate transformation of a likely meaningless number into conventional wisdom.

We all know that doctors make mistakes, sometimes fatal ones. That's not news. But when the National Academy of Sciences' Institute of Medicine waves the junk science wand over the unfortunate phenomenon, you get the headline,[145]

Medical Mistakes Blamed for Up to 98,000 Deaths a Year

Perceiving political gold in this statistic, some in Congress considered ways to reduce this "toll" through legislation.[146] Should Congress fiddle with our medical system on the basis of a statistic that can only be characterized as wrong? (Actual deaths from medical mistakes weren't identified or counted, and the margin of error for the "98,000" guessti-mate exceeded 100 percent.)

Statistics aren't science. They may be quantitative characteriza-tions of observations. They may be estimates from mathematical mod-els. In either case, statistics don't explain observations or validate models. Sometimes, statistics aren't even statistics.

Rule: Garbage In, Garbage Out

Statisticians aren't Rumpelstiltskins with calculators; they can't magi-cally spin bad data into science. A key consideration in evaluating a statistic is its underlying data quality.

Certified Mistakes

Consider, for example, death certificates. They're often used in epide-miologic investigations and for national statistics. You would think that physicians would always get the cause of death correct on death certificates. You would be wrong.

A study in the *Annals of Internal Medicine* recently reported that coronary heart disease may be overrepresented as a cause of death on death certificates.[147] Death certificates of the 2,683 decedents in the Framingham Heart Study attributed 24.3 percent more deaths to heart disease than did a panel of physicians reviewing the relevant medical records. For those at least 85 years of age, death certificates attributed 100 percent more deaths to heart disease than did the panel. Applying the 24.3 percent rate to the claimed 734,000 heart disease deaths annually in the United States, about 147,000 of these deaths may in fact be due to other causes.

The study's lead investigator, Daniel Levy, M.D., said, "If the cause of death is wrong, it is possible to miss fairly substantive relationships . . . and it could lead to inaccurate statistics."[148] Dorothy Rice, Ph.D., former director of the National Center for Health Statistics, said that the findings, "while not terribly surprising, are a little worri-some. . . . My concern is what cause of death did they understate."[149]

Self-Reported and Distorted

Bad data often arise from so-called self-reports. Many epidemiologic studies rely on data collected through interviews with study subjects. The studies usually rely exclusively on the word of the interviewee. No effort is made to verify responses.

A 1997 study by Harvard University researchers reported that study subjects "regularly" exposed to secondhand smoke had 90 percent more heart attacks than did those not "regularly" exposed.[150] But the data were self-reported and not verified by the researchers—even the data on whether someone ever had suffered a heart attack.

You might think that people could accurately report whether they've experienced a heart attack. But a recent study reported that as many as 40 percent of self-reported heart attacks are wrong.[151] It's enough to give you a coronary.

The Harvard researchers also relied on self-reports of smoking history. But many smokers fail to admit their smoking. It's a phenomenon called "smoker misclassification." Many people won't admit they smoke for insurance or social reasons. Misclassification rates can exceed 15 percent.[152]

It seems that it would be difficult to draw conclusions from study subjects who may erroneously report their own smoking status and whether they've even had a heart attack.

Bypass Bias

Another problem is the systematic distortion of data called "bias."

Studies on coronary heart disease (CHD) among postmenopausal women who use hormone replacement therapy (HRT) consistently report large, statistically significant decreases in CHD rates among HRT users. Many believe these studies indicate that HRT reduces risk of CHD. But as an editorial in the *Journal of the American Medical Association* recently stated:

> [HRT] users differ from nonusers in important respects; e.g., they are thinner, better educated, and more health-conscious. Substantial differ-

ences in their CHD risk factor profiles before commencing estrogen use could easily explain most of the subsequent differences in CHD rates. Women who use estrogen replacement therapy for a number of years are good compliers, and as such may have other attributes that predict better health. In addition, these women are or will be under closer medical supervision and, thus, have earlier diagnosis and treatment of health conditions, leading to a lower mortality than that among nonusers. On the other hand, women who cease estrogen replacement therapy frequently do so because of illness, which makes remaining users appear even healthier. These various biases are quite strong, and may account for most or even all of the apparent benefit for CHD in observational studies.[153]

The bias toward including women less prone to CHD in the studies of HRT makes the study result of reduced disease rates a foregone conclusion.

Bad data can't produce good statistics. Never give data the benefit of the doubt. Data must earn your respect.

Rule: Demand Definitions

"When I use a word, it means just what I choose it to mean—neither more nor less," said Humpty Dumpty in *Through the Looking Glass*. No doubt, he would be proud of how the junk science mob has taken his words to heart.

Former surgeon general Antonia Novello claimed in a May 1990 speech that 3,000 "kids" start smoking every day.[154] Since then, this statistic has become conventional wisdom. The statistic originated from researchers at the U.S. Centers for Disease Control and was published in the *Journal of the American Medical Association* in 1989.[155]

But if you read the actual study, you'll discover this acknowledgment: "For purposes of this analysis, only persons aged *20 years and older* are included" (emphasis added). Surely you understand why anti-smoking advocates don't claim "3,000 twenty-something kids start smoking every day."[156]

Advocates of gun control claim that 13 "kids" are killed by guns each day in America.[157] But this statistic includes people "ages 19 and under"—legal adults aged 18 and 19 are misleadingly counted as "kids."

Data from the National Center for Health Statistics indicate that, in 1997, there were 9 gunshot victims under one year of age, 75 gunshot victims between one and four years of age, and 546 gunshot victims between five and fourteen years of age. So if "kids" are considered those fourteen years of age and under, fewer than 2 "kids" per day are gunshot victims. There is no question that even 2 such deaths are tragic, but much less so than 13.

Look under the statistical rocks. You'll be surprised at what crawls out.

Rule: Statistics Don't Prove Cause and Effect

The EPA claimed in 1996 that fine particulate air pollution kills 20,000 Americans annually.[158] The basis for the estimate was a statistical study comparing death rates among geographic areas with varying levels of air pollution.

There were no clinical evaluations of any of the deaths included in the study. The researchers didn't know whether air pollution caused or contributed to any of the deaths. The researchers didn't have any idea of how much fine particulate air pollution any study subject inhaled. The statistic of "20,000 annual deaths" was essentially based on the assumption that "extra" deaths in areas with higher levels of air pollution were caused by the airborne fine particles. See the problem?

There's no cause-and-effect evidence behind the statistic. Even assuming there really was a difference in death rates among the geographic locations, there could be many explanations for the phenomenon. The researchers couldn't have ruled out these other explanations, much less have ruled in air pollution. The glaring information gaps should have precluded the study and the touted statistic from being considered scientific. But they didn't.

Statistical Malpractice

"Statistical Malpractice" by Bruce G. Charlton, M.D., of the University of Newcastle upon Tyne is one of the finest articles I've seen on the problem of treating statistics as science. Below are some key excerpts from this gem:

Science versus Statistics

There is a worrying trend in academic medicine which equates statistics with science, and sophistication in quantitative procedures with research excellence. The corollary of this trend is a tendency to look for answers to medical problems from people with expertise in mathematical manipulation and information technology, rather than from people with an understanding of disease and its causes.

Epidemiology [is a] main culprit, because statistical malpractice typically occurs when complex analytical techniques are combined with large data sets. The mystique of mathematics blended with the bewildering intricacies of big numbers makes a potent cocktail. . . .

The relationship between science and statistical analysis in medicine is quite simple: statistics is a tool of science which may or may not be useful for a given task. Indeed, the better the science, the less the need for complex analysis, and big databases are a sign not of rigor but of poor control. Basic scientists often quip that if statistics are needed, you should go back and do a better experiment. . . .

Science is concerned with *causes* but statistics is concerned with *correlations*. . . .

The prime concern of science is with minimizing systematic error (eliminating bias), while that of statistics is with minimizing random error (maximizing precision). Minimization of bias is a matter of controlling and excluding extraneous causes from observation and experiment so that the cause of interest may be isolated and characterized. . . . Maximization of precision, on the other hand, is the attempt to reveal the true magnitude of a variable which is being obscured by the "noise" [from the] limitations of measurement.

Science by Sleight-of-Hand

The root of most instances of statistical malpractice is the breaking of mathematical neutrality and the introduction of causal assumptions into the analysis without scientific grounds. This amounts to performing science by sleight-of-hand: the quickness of statistics deceives the mind. . . .

Practicing Science without a License

Statistical malpractice has an almost limitless potential for abuse, particularly in a context of the contemporary shift in emphasis away from curiosity-led science towards medical research driven by the imperatives of health policy and management. The difficulty is that statistical analysis is, apparently, applicable to any problem—just give it enough numbers and it will generate an answer. As a result, medicine has been deluged with more or less uninterpretable "answers" generated by heavyweight statistics operating on big databases of dubious validity. Such numerical manipulations cannot, in principle, do the work of hypothesis testing.

Statistical analysis has expanded beyond its legitimate realm of activity. The seductive offer of precision without the need for understanding is a snare to the incautious because exactitude is so often mistaken for explanation. Numerical technicians are now promoted to the status of general purpose experts on research methods, and the ultimate arbiters of the academic refereeing process. From the standpoint of medicine this is a mistake: statistics must be subordinate to the requirements of science, because human life and disease are consequences of a historical process of evolution which is not accessible to abstract mathematical analysis.[159]

Statistics can't prove cause-and-effect associations because they don't provide biological explanations. Without such explanations, statistical associations are hollow numbers.

Wanted: Biological Plausibility

A classic example of a statistical association backed up with biological plausibility is an incident of food poisoning that occurred in Italy in 1997.

Many students and faculty developed gastrointestinal illness after eating in a school cafeteria. The sick were 33 times more likely to have eaten the corn and tuna salad. Although an impressive statistic, without biological backup it's just a statistic. But the researchers matched the pathogen in stool samples with the salad from the caterer's kitchen. Such success is a rarity.

The absence of biological plausibility is fatal even to persistent statistics. Multiple epidemiologic studies report about a 50 percent increase in leukemia among children who live near electric power lines. But in its 1997 report on the potential health effects of electric and magnetic fields, a committee of the National Research Council noted that the absence of a biological explanation for the statistical association compelled it to conclude that "the current body of evidence does not show that exposure to [electric and magnetic fields] presents a human-health hazard."[160] The absence of biological plausibility electrocuted the statistical association.

Confound It!

Part of biological plausibility analysis is ruling out other factors that could be responsible for an observed statistical association.

On March 29, 2000, CBS News anchor Dan Rather announced, "A U.S. Air Force study of Vietnam veterans has found a strong link between exposure to the jungle defoliant Agent Orange and diabetes later in life." Compare Rather's terse and incomplete report with the *New York Times'* coverage:

> The study compared the health of 859 veterans of Operation Ranch Hand, who flew planes that sprayed the defoliant Agent Orange during the Vietnam War, to that of 1,232 who did not spray the chemical. There was no difference in the incidence of diabetes in the two groups— 16.9 percent of the Ranch Hand group was diabetic and 17 percent of the control group was diabetic.
>
> The diabetes effect only showed up when scientists looked at the levels of dioxin, the main chemical in Agent Orange, in the men's blood. After adjusting for factors like age and body fat levels, they concluded that the Ranch Hand participants with the lowest levels of dioxin in their blood had a 47 percent lower risk of diabetes than those with the highest levels of dioxin in their blood. . . .
>
> A major criticism of the Air Force study . . . has been that it is hard to sort out a dioxin effect from an effect of simply being overweight.
>
> Dioxin is stored in fat, so the fatter a person is, the higher his dioxin levels are likely to be. But the fatter someone is, the more likely he is to develop diabetes. The question scientists asked was, is the effect due to dioxin or to obesity?
>
> "We know diabetes is highly related to body fat, and so is dioxin," [the lead researcher] said. "That's why these diabetes findings are so

difficult to interpret. People are concerned that we haven't done the right body fat adjustment."[161]

A link between dioxin and diabetes is not supported by other epidemiologic studies.[162]

Smoking Out a Confounder

Smoking Ban Boosted Health of Bartenders, Study Reports

was a *Los Angeles Times* headline on December 9, 1998. The article continued:

> San Francisco bartenders showed dramatic improvements in lung health within two months after the January implementation of California's indoor smoking ban, UC San Francisco researchers report today.
> Bartenders were exposed to unusually high levels of secondhand smoke before the ban—about four to six times the level found in other workplaces.
> Examining 53 bartenders before and after the ban was implemented, Dr. Mark D. Eisner and his colleagues at UC San Francisco found that 59% of those reporting respiratory problems, such as wheezing, shortness of breath and morning coughing, were symptom-free less than two months after the ban began.
> Moreover, they report in today's Journal of the American Medical Assn., 78% of those with eye, nose or throat irritation were also symptom-free.
> "That's a pretty big change over a short period of time," Eisner said. Although the number of people studied is relatively small, the results are considered statistically significant. . . .
> In an editorial in the same issue of the journal, Dr. Ronald M. Davis of the Henry Ford Health System in Detroit called for further smoking bans across the country.

But of the study's 53 bartenders, 24 smoked—smoking is a risk factor for lung illnesses. And what the *Times* didn't report was key information describing when the data were collected:

> From December 1 to 31, 1997, we interviewed and performed spirometry on participating bartenders in their workplaces (bar or tavern). Follow-

up interviews and spirometry were performed from February 1 to 28, 1998, to evaluate changes in symptoms or lung function following the institution of smoke-free bars.[163]

Notice anything? Bartenders were interviewed about their respiratory health in the middle of flu season and then reinterviewed when flu season was over. Perhaps this is why the study authors were compelled to note at the end of their study, "Confounding by personal smoking and [upper respiratory infections] could potentially explain the observed improvement in respiratory health."[164]

But the *Times* apparently wasn't interested in the headline, "Bartenders Get Flu and Recover, Study Says." Such a headline would also not go far in justifying a smoking ban.

No Statistical Wand

Beware, though. Just because researchers claim to have eliminated confounders doesn't mean they have. Unfortunately, most researchers try to eliminate confounders only through statistics. As you have no doubt committed to memory by now, statistics are not science. Here's what Dr. Charlton had to say about statistical adjustment for confounders:

> [Science by sleight of hand] commonly happens when statistical adjustments . . . are performed to remove the effects of confounding variables. These are manoeuvers by which data sets are recalculated (e.g., by stratified or multivariate analysis) in an attempt to eliminate the consequences of uncontrolled "interfering" variables which distort the causal relationship under study. For instance, standardizing for age in a study of smoking and cancer may involve imbalances in the population age structure of smokers and non-smokers being "corrected" using statistical manipulations.
>
> There are, however, no statistical rules by which confounders can be identified, and the process of adjustment involves making quantitative causal assumptions based upon secondary analysis of the data base in question. This may not matter much if the objective is simply to provide a summary statistic for the purpose of comparison, but is illegitimate as part of a scientific enquiry because it amounts to a tacit attempt to test two hypotheses using only a simple set of observations.

Adjustment is therefore, implicitly, a way of modeling the magnitude of a causal process in order to subtract its effects from the data. However, modeling is not mathematically neutral and involves importing assumptions—an activity which requires to be justified for each case. Before statistical "correction" is applied, the quantitative model describing the causal relationship between age, smoking and cancer should itself be replicated by testing against other independent sources of data. Yet this stage is typically omitted, presumably because adjustment is considered to be a purely mathematical, and therefore neutral, procedure.

This question of modeling provides a useful distinction between statistics and science. A scientific model is built up from theories concerning causal assumptions, and has itself the character of a hypothesis that brings with it the need for replication. By contrast, statistical models are fundamentally *post hoc* and atheoretical, being derived from data sets by mathematical algorithms, such as constructing a "best fit" curve. . . . A statistical model does not, therefore, advance understanding, being of the nature of a summary of observations rather than a theory of how the world is: validity is derived wholly from the data fed into it.[165]

The bottom line: There is no "statistical wand" that can be waved to remove confounders. Statistical procedures cannot make up for the lack of information in the data.[166] What would be really useful, though, is an "honesty wand."

Smoke and Mirrors

Researchers aren't necessarily going to tell you what confounders weren't considered, why they weren't considered, and what the possible impacts on their statistical associations would be.

Second-Hand Smoke Linked to Breast Cancer

headlined the *Toronto Star* in March 2000. The article continued:

Alarming new research from Health Canada suggests exposure to second-hand smoke may increase the risk of breast cancer, and the longer the exposure, the higher the risk.

Conducted by researchers at Health Canada's Laboratory Centre for Disease Control, the study was published yesterday in the scientific journal Cancer Causes and Control.

"This speaks to the need for protecting our children from the harmful effects of second-hand smoke and the need to find ways to discourage young girls from taking up smoking," said Dr. Barbara Whylie, the Canadian Cancer Society's director of medical affairs and cancer control.

The study compared 1,420 women newly diagnosed with breast cancer to approximately 1,400 women who did not have the disease, Health Canada reports.

Researchers found the risk of breast cancer in premenopausal women increased by 100 per cent if they were exposed to second-hand smoke for a long time—around 20 years.

For women over 50 years old who had experienced menopause, a couple of decades of exposure to second-hand smoke increased their breast-cancer risk by 30 per cent.[167]

But the media missed, and the researchers didn't volunteer, the study's stunning irregularity.

The 4,755 women studied were interviewed about health history relevant to breast cancer risk, including age at first menstruation, age at first pregnancy, number of live births, and other potential risk factors for breast cancer.[168] Only a small subset of women was asked about family history of breast cancer and history of benign breast disease—two other well-known breast cancer risk factors.

Among the women in the subset, the researchers reported that having a mother or sister with breast cancer quadrupled the risk of breast cancer. A history of benign breast disease reportedly increased the risk of breast cancer by 500 percent. Oddly enough, the researchers didn't factor family history or history of benign disease into their touted results.

In contrast, other recent research examining potential relationships between lifestyle factors (such as diet and exercise) and breast cancer published in prominent medical journals, including the *Journal of the National Cancer Institute*[169] and the *New England Journal of Medicine*,[170] considered family history of breast cancer and history of benign breast disease. Was this simple oversight that of the researchers or of *Cancer Causes and Control*, the journal publishing the study?

The researchers knew these risk factors were important—they collected data on them. If the results couldn't be adjusted for all key risk factors, this deficiency should have been flagged. Not adjusting the results for family history and history of benign disease is not even alluded to in the study's discussion section. The fine print must be carefully reviewed to discover the omission.

Researchers aren't infallible or beyond reproach. This is why scientific journals have editorial and peer review. The editor of *Cancer Causes and Control* is Harvard University's Graham Colditz, author of numerous papers on breast cancer. Colditz has not only studied family history as a breast cancer risk factor, but also factors it into his studies of other breast cancer risk factors.[171] How could Colditz have overlooked the omission of the Health Canada researchers? Or was he thinking that everyone else would? The media certainly did.

And that's the true value of statistics to junk science. The junk scientist bet is that you won't notice the statistical sleight of hand—or even try to find it. But you should try. The fraud's on you.

LESSON 4:
EPIDEMIOLOGY IS STATISTICS

Statistics are used by people who have no proof.

—Anonymous

A LEADING EPIDEMIOLOGY textbook defines epidemiology as study

> concerned with the patterns of disease occurrence in human populations
> and the factors that influence these patterns. Epidemiologists are primar-
> ily interested in the occurrence of disease as categorized by time, place
> and persons. They try to determine whether there has been an increase
> or decrease of the disease over the years, whether one geographical
> area has a higher frequency of disease than another, and whether the
> characteristics of persons with a particular disease or condition distin-
> guish them from those without it.[172]

So what do epidemiologists actually do? Statistics! That's the essence
of epidemiology. And you remember what statistics aren't, right?

It's not that epidemiology isn't a useful tool in studying disease.
It is. But it has limitations.

There are four basic types (or "designs") of epidemiologic studies
for Junk Science Judo purposes:

- clinical trials,
- cohort studies,

- case-control studies, and
- ecologic studies.

Each design has a particular utility. All attempt to produce the same key result: a statistical association between an exposure of interest and a disease of interest.

The different study designs require slightly different statistical analyses, but the real substantive difference is the level of confidence each design confers on the associations that are developed. The difference in confidence is due to the level of control the epidemiologist has over the study data.

Clinical trials differ fundamentally from cohort, case-control, and ecologic studies because they are "experimental" in nature. In clinical trials, researchers assign exposures to study subjects. Cohort, case-control, and ecologic studies, on the other hand, are "observational"— the researchers can only observe the outcomes of exposures that are out of their control.

Because greater researcher control over data tends to produce more reliable data, statistical associations calculated from clinical trials tend to be more reliable. They remain statistics, but they tend to be more reliable statistics.

Let's go over some simplified, real-life examples of the different types of studies and the statistical associations they produce.

Clinical Trials

Clinical trials are typically used to test the efficacy of medical treatments. You may run into clinical trial–based junk science when researchers tout new medical treatments.

Study: Estrogen Substitute Lowers Risk of Breast Cancer

the Associated Press reported on June 15, 1999. The article continued:

> An estrogen substitute used to prevent brittle bones in women
> who are past menopause reduces the risk of breast cancer dramatically,

a study found. The three-year study of 7,705 women found a 76 percent lower risk of breast cancer among those taking raloxifene compared with those given a placebo.

The AP reported on a clinical trial in which the researchers assigned study subjects to take either raloxifene or a placebo.[173] The women were followed for an average of 40 months.

At the end of the clinical trial, the researchers reported that, among the 2,576 women who took the placebo, 27 cases of invasive breast cancer occurred; among the 5,129 women who took raloxifene, 13 cases of invasive breast cancer occurred. These results are presented in Table 4.1.

To determine the apparent efficacy of raloxifene, the researchers compared the rates of breast cancer among the treatment and placebo groups. This rate comparison—or "statistical association"—is called the relative risk. The relative risk of breast cancer among women taking raloxifene in this study was

$$\text{Relative risk} = \frac{\text{Rate of breast cancer among women receiving raloxifene}}{\text{Rate of breast cancer among women receiving placebo}}$$

or

$$\text{Relative risk} = \frac{13 \div 5{,}129}{27 \div 2{,}576} = 0.24$$

The relative risk of 0.24 means there was 24 percent as much breast cancer among the raloxifene group as among the placebo group. It can also be said (as in the AP report, above) there was 76 percent

Table 4.1: Breast Cancer and Raloxifene

Drug	Breast Cancers	Subjects
Raloxifene	13	5,129
Placebo	27	2,576

less breast cancer among the raloxifene group than among the placebo group. But the relative risk does not prove that raloxifene caused the difference in breast cancer rates among the two groups; it merely indicates that there was a difference in breast cancer rates.

Why doesn't this study prove that raloxifene reduces breast cancer risk? The researchers did not show that raloxifene actually prevented any breast cancers that otherwise would have occurred. It is possible that the reported difference in breast cancer rates between the two groups is due to some unknown risk factor for breast cancer not considered or controlled, or even due to chance.

Raloxifene manufacturer Eli Lilly & Co. wanted to use the results of the clinical trial to market raloxifene as a breast cancer prevention drug. But a federal judge issued an injunction against such marketing, ruling that the study did not prove that raloxifene prevented breast cancer.

Cohort Studies

A cohort study is an observational study in which the researcher has no control over the exposure of interest. Instead, the researcher observes only health outcomes potentially associated with the exposure. To conduct a cohort study, a researcher will identify a group of people to study, obtain relevant information about the study subjects, and then follow them for a period of time to see who dies or develops the health condition of interest.

Study Says Caffeine Might Protect against Parkinson's Disease

the Associated Press reported on May 23, 2000. The article continued:

> An intriguing new study suggests coffee may prevent Parkinson's disease. How a product that makes people jittery could keep them from getting a disease that gives them tremors is a paradox not examined in the study of 8,004 Japanese-American men in Hawaii.
>
> But the researchers said the benefits are probably due to caffeine— apparently the more, the better—and they suggest some theories about how it might work. . . .

The study found that men who didn't drink coffee were five times more likely to develop Parkinson's than those who drank the most—4½ to 5 ½ 6-ounce cups a day. Non-coffee drinkers were two to three times more likely to get the disease than men who drank 4 ounces to four cups a day. . . .

The researchers examined data from the ongoing Honolulu Heart Program. Participants—age 53 on average when the study began—were asked about coffee consumption at the outset in 1965 and again in 1971. The researchers then measured Parkinson's disease rates from 1991 to 1996. The disease developed in 102 men.

Among the 1,286 men who weren't coffee drinkers, the researchers counted 32 men with Parkinson's disease.[174] Among the 959 men in the group with the highest level of coffee consumption (more than 3 cups per day), the researchers counted 4 men with Parkinson's disease. These counts are presented in Table 4.2.

The statistical association of interest is the relative risk of Parkinson's disease among those who drank no coffee:

$$\text{Relative risk} = \frac{\text{Rate of PD among men with no coffee intake}}{\text{Rate of PD among men with high coffee intake}}$$

or

$$\text{Relative risk} = \frac{32 \div 1{,}286}{4 \div 959} = 5.9$$

As reported by the AP, the population of men who drank no coffee had roughly five times more Parkinson's disease than the population of men who drank a lot of coffee. Another way of looking at this statistical

Table 4.2: Coffee and Parkinson's Disease

	Cases of PD	No PD	Total
High coffee intake	4	955	959
No coffee intake	32	1,254	1,286

association is to turn it upside down. The relative risk of Parkinson's disease among those who consumed a lot of coffee is

$$\text{Relative risk} = \frac{\text{Rate of PD among men with high coffee intake}}{\text{Rate of PD among men with no coffee intake}}$$

or

$$\text{Relative risk} = \frac{4 \div 959}{32 \div 1{,}286} = 0.17$$

This result means that the population of coffee drinkers had 17 percent as much—or 83 percent less—Parkinson's disease as the population of non–coffee drinkers. This is the same result as reported in the Associated Press article, but it looks at a potential "protective" effect of coffee drinking as opposed to the "risk" from not drinking coffee.   Despite its apparently impressive results, this study also has significant limitations.

The reported relative risk is again just a statistical comparison of the two groups. The researchers did not prove that coffee consumption was the cause of the observed difference in rates of Parkinson's disease. But worse than in the clinical trial example, the researchers don't really know how much coffee any subject consumed.

Data on coffee consumption were collected only twice—in 1965 and 1971. The researchers assumed that the level of coffee consumption reported at those times was the level of coffee consumption throughout the length of the study—about 30 years. Compare this guesstimate of coffee consumption with the clinical trial example, where the researchers knew precisely how much raloxifene each treated woman received.

You can already see the steep decline in data quality from clinical trial to cohort study. It gets even worse in case-control and ecologic studies.

Case-Control Studies

Case-control studies are cohort studies in reverse. Cohort studies start with disease-free subjects and follow them into the future to see if those with the exposure of interest develop disease. Case-control studies, in contrast, start with study subjects with the disease of interest and try to examine their history to see whether an exposure of interest is statistically associated with the disease of interest. Cohort studies are prospective; case-control studies are retrospective.

You can already see how the data quality of case-control studies slips in comparison with that of cohort studies. In the cohort study, above, subjects were asked in 1965 about their *current* level of coffee consumption. Had that study been a case-control study, the subjects would have been asked in 1996 about their coffee consumption in 1965. Could you remember how much coffee you drank 30 years ago?

Here's an example of the case-control design at work involving a recent study reporting an association between environmental tobacco smoke (ETS) and head/neck cancer.[175] The researchers identified 155 subjects who had head/neck cancer (cases) and 166 subjects who did not (controls). Of the 155 cases, 145 said they had been exposed to ETS and 10 said they had not been exposed to ETS. Of the 166 controls, 139 said they had been exposed to ETS and 27 said they had not been exposed to ETS. The counts are presented in Table 4.3.

In case-control studies, the statistical association technically is called an "odds ratio." But for ease of discussion, we will refer to it as "relative risk."

Table 4.3: ETS and Cancer

Exposure to ETS	Cases	Controls
Ever exposed to ETS	145	139
Never exposed to ETS	10	27

The data collected from the cases and controls indicate that the relative risk of head/neck cancer among those exposed to ETS is

$$\text{Relative risk} = \frac{\text{Ratio of ETS exposure among the cases}}{\text{Ratio of ETS exposure among the controls}}$$

or

$$\text{Relative risk} = \frac{145 \div 10}{139 \div 27} = 2.8$$

The interpretation of the relative risk is that the cases were 2.8 times more likely than the controls to have been exposed to ETS.

But as in the examples of the clinical trial and cohort study, the researchers demonstrated only a statistical difference between the groups compared. They do not actually know that ETS is the cause of the difference. The difference between the two groups could be due to some unknown factor correlating with the treatment group or chance. What makes the relative risk from the case-control study less reliable than a relative risk from a cohort study is the data quality.

Data on exposure to ETS were collected by interviewing the study subjects. Study subjects who said they were "occasionally" or "regularly" exposed to ETS at home or work were classified as "ever exposed" to ETS. Those classified as "never exposed" reportedly had not even "occasionally" been exposed to ETS in the home or at work. But isn't this classification system rather "loosey-goosey"?

What are "occasional" and "regular" exposures to ETS? Is exposure once per week, every week, "occasional" or "regular"? How did study subjects distinguish between infrequent exposures to a relatively high level of ETS and frequent exposures to relatively low levels of ETS? And who can credibly claim that she has never been exposed to environmental tobacco smoke?

Moreover, everyone knows about the association between smoking and cancer. If you were diagnosed with cancer and were asked about past exposures to ETS, wouldn't you do a better job of racking your memory than if you weren't diagnosed with cancer? Probably. Epidemiologists call this phenomenon "recall bias." It doesn't imply dishonesty, only memory problems. Too often, epidemiologists who know about recall bias ignore it.

The average age of this study population is about 60 years. Weren't smoking rates relatively high during the 1950s, 1960s, and 1970s— a time when these study subjects were likely in the workforce? There weren't very many restrictions on smoking back then. The researchers did not ask about exposure to ETS in social situations.

The burden of case-control study researchers is that they must accept the "exposure" data at face value and be satisfied with not really knowing who was exposed to what. The alternative is not to have a study. You, on the other hand, don't have to accept case-control nonsense. Remember: garbage in, garbage out.

But you don't have to take my word. Here's what Harvard University epidemiologists had to say in the context of homocysteine, the latest fad in risk factors for heart disease. On the basis of case-control studies, researchers have reported that moderately elevated levels of homocysteine are associated with moderate increases in rates of heart disease. Cohort studies, on the other hand, report little or no association between homocysteine levels and heart disease. The Harvard researchers wrote:

> In case-control studies, differences in the recall or ascertainment of exposure history according to disease status are always an important potential source of bias, whereas, prospective studies have the major advantage of collecting blood specimens before any relevant clinical events have occurred. Thus, the temporal relationship between elevated homocysteine levels and [cardiovascular disease] risk is more clearly defined in [cohort] studies than in . . . case-control studies. In addition, information on [other potential risk factors for heart disease] can be collected before the occurrence of relevant clinical events in [cohort] studies.[176]

They concluded that homocysteine may be just an artifact, not a cause, of atherosclerosis.

Remember: Case-control means out of control.

Ecologic Studies

At the bottom of the epidemiologic barrel is the so-called ecologic study design. Ecologic studies are so unreliable that they have a specially named deficiency—the "ecologic fallacy."

Unlike clinical trials, cohort studies, and case-control studies—all of which use data collected about individual study subjects—ecologic studies use only data collected about populations. An ecologic study might involve attempting to associate the difference in disease rates between geographically distinct communities with some "exposure" factor associated with one of the communities.

Weed Killer Ecology

Here's an example of the ecologic design at work, a study attempting to link a class of weed killers (chlorophenoxy herbicides) with increased cancer rates.[177]

The study collected data on cancer incidence and wheat production for the counties of four wheat-producing states (Minnesota, North Dakota, South Dakota, and Montana). A sample of the data collected for white women is presented in Table 4.4.

The data indicate that the cancer death rate is 1 percent higher and 5 percent higher in counties with medium and high levels of wheat acreage, respectively, than in counties with low levels of wheat acreage. So what do these data have to do with herbicides? That's a good question.

Table 4.4: Wheat and Cancer

| | Wheat Acreage per County | | |
	Low	Medium	High
Population	349,660	160,200	134,105
Number of cancers (1980–89)	7,824	4,161	3,574
Cancer mortality rate (age adjusted)	1.00	1.01	1.05

The researcher's theory is that because more than 90 percent of spring and durum wheat is treated with herbicides, wheat production is a surrogate measure for exposure to herbicides. Therefore, higher cancer rates in geographic areas with more wheat farming implicate herbicides as the cause, according to the researcher.

The problem, of course, is that the researcher collected no data from any individuals on actual exposures to herbicides or other cancer risk factors. So no data link individual exposures to herbicides with cancer incidence.

Not only does the researcher not have any control over the data, the researcher doesn't even really know what the data are! This is the so-called ecologic fallacy—communities may differ in many factors, and one or more of those may be the underlying reason for the difference in observed disease and death rates.

The ecologic method might be useful in providing researchers with ideas for future research, but nothing more.

Ecologic by Any Name

You should be aware of "stealth" ecologic studies, which mix the ecologic study design with either the cohort or case-control design and then are misleadingly referred to as cohort or case-control studies.

Study Ties Fouled Air to High Urban Death Rates

reported the *New York Times* on December 9, 1993. The article continued:

> A study of six cities has found that air pollution, even in areas that meet Federal air quality standards, can shorten people's lives.
>
> The study, to be published Thursday in the *New England Journal of Medicine*, says air pollution can shorten lives by up to two years. It also says the smallest particles, like those from automobile exhausts and smokestacks, seem mostly responsible. . . . The findings suggest that urban air pollution standards in the United States may not be sufficiently stringent.

The study said mortality rates from lung cancer, lung disease and heart disease were 26 percent higher in Steubenville, Ohio, the most polluted area studied, than in Portage, Wis., which was the least polluted. The air in Steubenville had, on average, three times more fine particles of pollution than that in Portage, but particle pollution levels did not exceed Federal limits.

The authors of the so-called Six-City Study collected data on death rates and air pollution levels in six cities.[178] The data are summarized in Table 4.5.

Compared with Portage, the city with the lowest level of fine particulate air pollution, the five cities with higher air pollution rates reportedly have higher death rates. What's the problem?

The researchers called this study design a "cohort study" and, in some respects, it is. The researchers collected some data on individual study subjects from 1975 through 1991. The problem, though, is that no data on individual exposures to air pollution were collected.

The researchers instead used area-wide measurements of fine particles for each city. The researchers assumed that study subjects living in Steubenville, Ohio, were exposed to higher levels of air pollution than were those living in Portage, Wisconsin. But this is not necessarily true.

Table 4.5: Death Rates and Air Pollution

	City					
	Portage	Topeka	Watertown	Harriman	St. Louis	Steubenville
Subjects	1,631	1,239	1,336	1,258	1,296	1,351
Deaths	232	156	248	222	281	291
Death rate[a]	10.73	9.68	12.47	12.45	15.86	16.24
Fine particles[b]	11.0	12.5	14.9	20.8	19.0	29.6
Relative risk	1.00	1.01	1.17	1.07	1.14	1.26

[a]Death rates are shown in deaths per 1,000 person-years.
[b]Fine particles are measured in millionths of a gram per cubic meter.

Exposure to air pollution depends on many factors, including where study subjects lived and worked in relation to the air monitors, time spent outside versus inside, and the reliability of the monitors. The researchers, in fact, had no control over individual exposures to fine particles. The exposure data are clearly ecologic in nature and so the study is subject to the ecologic fallacy.

So why did the researchers call this a "cohort study"? The *New York Times* reported, "The new study, under the direction of Douglas Dockery of Harvard University's School of Public Health, tried to overcome the shortcomings of earlier studies." The "shortcoming" of the earlier studies was that they were ecologic studies. It seems that Dockery overcame this shortcoming by labeling the Six-City Study a "cohort" study.

An Epidemiologic Success Story

I don't want to you to lose faith completely in epidemiologic studies, though. They can be useful. Here's an example of what epidemiology is supposed to be all about. It's even a case-control study, at that.

On May 21, 1997, 292 students and staff at two primary schools in northern Italy were hospitalized with gastrointestinal illnesses. All the students and staff had eaten at school cafeterias served by the same caterer. The researchers interviewed 2,189 persons, 82 percent of whom had eaten at the cafeterias. Of these, 1,566 reported symptoms of gastrointestinal illness. The researchers interviewed the students and staff about what they ate. Table 4.6 shows the results for the pasta with olive oil served in the cafeteria

Based on the data collected from students and staff, the relative risk of being ill after consuming the pasta with olive oil is

Table 4.6: Pasta and Illness

	No. Ill	No. Not Ill
Ate the pasta	1,041	525
Did not eat the pasta	417	206

$$\text{Relative risk} = \frac{\text{Ratio of pasta eaters to those with illness}}{\text{Ratio of pasta eaters to those without illness}}$$

or

$$\text{Relative risk} = \frac{1{,}041 \div 417}{525 \div 206} = 0.98$$

Since 0.98 is essentially the same as 1.0, there was no difference in rates of pasta consumption among the cases and controls. The pasta wasn't the culprit.

The researchers looked at the data for Parmesan cheese, summarized in Table 4.7.

Based on the data collected from students and staff, the relative risk of being ill after consuming the Parmesan cheese is

$$\text{Relative risk} = \frac{1{,}025 \div 401}{541 \div 222} = 1.05$$

Once again, 1.05 is so close to 1.0, the researchers concluded the Parmesan cheese wasn't the culprit.

Finally, the researchers looked at the data for the corn and tuna salad, summarized in Table 4.8.

Table 4.7: Cheese and Illness

	No. Ill	No. Not Ill
Ate Parmesan cheese	1,025	541
Did not eat Parmesan cheese	401	222

Table 4.8: Corn and Tuna Salad and Illness

	No. Ill	No. Not Ill
Ate corn and tuna salad	1,514	291
Did not eat corn and tuna salad	52	332

Based on the data collected from students and staff, the relative risk of being ill after consuming the corn and tuna salad is

$$\text{Relative risk} = \frac{1{,}514 \div 52}{291 \div 332} = 33.22$$

Wow! Those who were ill were 33 times more likely to have eaten the corn and tuna salad. The researchers started to think the corn and tuna salad was responsible for the food poisoning. But because statistics aren't science, the researchers need to confirm their results scientifically.

The bacterium *Listeria monocytogenes* was isolated from 123 of 141 stool samples collected from those who were hospitalized. *Listeria monocytogenes* was also isolated from the caterer's sample of the salad and from specimens collected at the catering plant. All the *Listeria* samples collected were found to be genetically identical. Case (-control study) closed.

This is a model epidemiologic study because the study design was well suited to the problem—an unusual outbreak of food poisoning among a well-defined population over a limited period of time. Strong statistical analysis backed up with sound laboratory work solved the problem.

The epidemiologic study does not work well where researchers are faced with common health endpoints occurring among the general population over long periods of time. Such studies tend to produce flaky statistical associations that cannot be scientifically supported.

The "Black Box"

What's the bottom line on epidemiology? It's a good statistical tool for the study of certain disease patterns—but too often, it's misused. I like the way the late Petr Skrabanek described the misuse of epidemiology in his article "The Emptiness of the Black Box," excerpted below:

> The "black box" strategy is a current paradigm of epidemiologic research, better described by the term "risk factor epidemiology." In the hope of unraveling causes of diseases, associations are sought between disease

and various "exposures." "Black box" is an untested postulate linking the exposure and the disease in a causal sequence. An association, by itself a fortuitous finding, is thus converted, by logical sleight-of-hand, into a causal link. The causal mechanism remains unknown ("black"), but its existence is implied ("box"). Advocates of this strategy see it as a "unique virtue" of epidemiology [footnote omitted] and the source of "the most important findings [of cancer causation] thus far. . . . The 'black box' strategy looks at the cancers that people chiefly die of and then looks for populations (defined by country or county of residence, by dietary, drinking or smoking habits, religion, occupation, or reproduction, and by many other aspects of people's lifestyle or environment) which differ in death rates from these cancers to determine what seem to be the chief manipulable determinants [= causes] of today's cancers." [footnote omitted]

Its detractors believe that this strategy is an embarrassing liability. [footnotes omitted] As there are no underlying hypotheses for this kind of "research," beyond a general feeling that "diseases of civilization" are caused by civilization, the method is based on "stabs in the dark". . . . by which various "biologically vague but important circumstances," such as lifestyle, are randomly linked to various chronic diseases. . . .

The aim of science is to find universal laws governing the world around us and within us; it is about dismantling the "black box." It is doubtful that anything is ever discovered by "stabs in the dark." In science, at least, one proceeds from an interesting problem, embedded within a larger body of systematized knowledge, toward its solution or rejection. Reasoning such as "the existence of cars is associated with car accidents; *ergo*, let us ban cars and there will be no more car accidents," may be relevant for public health, but it is not science.

Black box epidemiology disparages understanding. It takes shortcuts to be able to issue "warnings," which because of the studied "exposures," often overlap with exhortations of politically correct moralists. . . .

The futility of black box research can be demonstrated by the example of the endless stream of studies attempting to implicate coffee drinking as the "cause" of various diseases. As the United States imports some 3 billion pounds of coffee annually, its ubiquitous consumption might have been of public health importance, if and only if there were a shred of evidence that the various associations reported in the epidemiologic literature are truly causal. For the past 30 years, a debate has been going on whether coffee drinking is causally linked to coronary heart disease. Three different positions have been taken: the risk of coronary heart disease is increased, not changed, or decreased. The impasse is unlikely to be resolved by further case-control studies. The same can be said about the associations between coffee drinking and bladder cancer: a recent review of 35 case-control studies, spanning 20 years of wasted effort failed to find any clinically important association [footnote omitted].[179]

If all this is Greek to you, the following example should help clarify the perils of the statistical nature of epidemiology.

You Bet Your Life
In October 1999, NBC's *Today* show reported,

> Important health news this morning. Women who exercise at least an hour a day may reduce their risk of breast cancer by 20 percent. That's according to one of the largest studies ever conducted on the subject. Exercise lowers the level of estrogen in a woman's body, and researchers believe that high estrogen levels increase the chance of—chances of cancer.[180]

Researchers studied data on physical activity from 85,364 women and the 3,137 cases of breast cancer occurring among the women.[181] They reported that there was about 20 percent less breast cancer among the women who claimed to engage in moderate or vigorous physical activity for seven or more hours per week compared with those who said they engaged in such physical activity for less than one hour per week.[182]

Let's assume for the sake of argument that the study result is "true"—that the population of women who exercised at least one hour per day had 20 percent less breast cancer. Let's further assume that of every 1,000 women, 30 will get breast cancer over the course of a lifetime. But which 30? No one knows. Breast cancer is not predictable with anything approaching certainty—even among women with recognized risk factors.

Then among a population of 1,000 women who exercise daily, 24 women instead of 30 women will develop breast cancer (i.e., 30 less 20 percent). But which 24? As before, no one knows.

So what's the benefit of exercise, in terms of breast cancer risk, for an individual woman? Not much. Even an exercising woman must remain vigilant about breast cancer—early detection of the disease dramatically increases the chances of survival. An exercising woman could just as easily be one of the 24 as one of the 30 who will develop breast cancer.

The potential breast cancer benefit of all women exercising—if true—shows up only on a population—or statistical—basis. And relying on statistics could turn you into one.

LESSON 5:
SIZE MATTERS

*Like other occult techniques of divination, the
statistical method has a private jargon deliberately
contrived to obscure its methods from
non-practitioners.*

—G. O. Ashley

SIZE DOES MATTER—at least in epidemiology.

With the general exception of clinical trials, the data collected
and analyzed by "risk factor" epidemiologists can be kind of goofy.
As a consequence, there is a general rule of thumb about epidemiologic studies.

Rule: Epidemiology Is for High Rates of Rare Diseases

A classic example of this rule is the statistical association between
cigarette smoking and lung cancer. Lung cancer is a rare disease,
striking perhaps 1 of every 10,000 nonsmokers over the course of a
lifetime. But U.S. smokers have rates of lung cancer that are 10 to 20
times greater than those of nonsmokers—a relatively high rate of a
rare disease.

How high is high? How rare is rare? There's good news and bad news. First the bad news. Specific guidelines for what is a "rare" disease don't exist. That's something that needs to be considered case by case.

Generally, though, illnesses like heart disease and "all cancers combined" aren't easy to assess through epidemiology because they are common diseases. About one-half of all U.S. men and one-third of U.S. women will get cancer during their lifetimes, according to the American Cancer Society. Cardiovascular disease is the leading cause of death for both men and women, according to the American Heart Association.

The good news is that specific guidelines exist for determining what is a "high" rate of disease. All you need do is consider the size of the relative risk. If a relative risk is really large or really small, there may be something to the statistic after all—no guarantees, though. Statistics aren't science.

Rule: Ignore Relative Risks between 0.50 and 2.0

A relative risk of 1.0 means there is no difference in rate of disease between two study populations. A relative risk of 2.0 means that the study population with the exposure of interest has double the rate of disease (100 percent more) than the nonexposed population. A relative risk of 3.0 means the rate is three times as high (200 percent more), 4.0 means four times as high (300 percent more), and so forth.

Increases in relative risk on the order of 100 percent and less— i.e., relative risks of between 1.0 and 2.0—should be viewed suspiciously. The esteemed epidemiologist Ernst Wynder even said that relative risks under 3.0 are suspect.[183] Given the nature of the epidemiologic method and the quality of the data, such small differences could easily be explained by the quality of the data. A 100 percent increase in risk may sound like a lot, but in epidemiology, it's not.

Decreases in relative risk on the order of 50 percent or less— i.e., relative risks between 0.50 and 1.0—should be viewed with suspicion. Why 0.50 and 1.0? If you think about it, a 50 percent decline from 1.0 is the same as a 100 percent increase from 0.50. These small increases and decreases in relative risk are called "weak statistical associations" or just "weak associations."

None of this is to say that it's impossible for a small change in relative risk to be valid. But I can't think of a single example—not one.

Sir Austin Bradford Hill, the dean of modern epidemiology, laid out the criteria for evaluating epidemiologic studies in his famous address to the Royal Society of Medicine in 1965. Hill drew the line at a relative risk of 2.0.

> First upon my list I would put the strength of the association. . . . Prospective inquiries into smoking have shown that the death rate from cancer of the lung in cigarette smokers is one to ten times the rate in non-smokers. . . . On the other hand, the death rate from coronary thrombosis in smokers is no more than twice, possibly less, the death rate in non-smokers. Though there is good evidence to support causation, it is surely much easier in this case to think of some features of life that may go hand-in-hand with smoking—features that might conceivably be the real underlying cause or, at least, an important contributor, whether it be lack of exercise, nature of diet or other factors.[184]

About weak statistical associations, Wynder commented,

> Today we find numerous publications with relative risks of less than 2 that do not discuss the extent to which [causal criteria for epidemiology] fit with their conclusions. Studies reporting on the relation of alcohol to breast cancer, for example, generally do not consider that the global distribution of alcohol consumption does not correlate with incidence of breast cancer. Epidemiologic studies on diesel exhaust exposure and its relation to lung cancer do not report that positive animal studies were based on a major overload of the rat's pulmonary system. Investigations suggesting that cigarette smoking relates to cancer of the cervix do not report that the marked increase in smoking in women is inconsistent with the steep reduction in cervical cancer rates. Usually, inconsistencies between studies, which often exist in reports of weak associations, are not fully presented. In short, as we determine whether a relation is causative, the criteria of judgment including consistency, time trends, dose response, and biologic plausibility are often neglected. We should more diligently consider these criteria. We should not rush to judgment

about a causative implication when in fact the word "association" ought to be used. Here again, we recognize that the wish bias tends to lead the investigator to conclude that a reported association is causative or to give that implication.[185]

Get the idea? If not, there's the story about the studies claiming to link abortion with breast cancer.

Abortion Contortion

Researchers recently reported a 30 percent increase in breast cancer (a relative risk of 1.3) among women who had had abortions as compared with women who hadn't had abortions.[186] This may sound like a large risk, but remember our rule about the size of relative risks. If you've forgotten, here's the public health establishment to remind you:

- The National Cancer Institute issued a special press release about abortion and breast cancer stating, "In epidemiologic research, relative risks of less than 2 are considered small and usually difficult to interpret. Such increases may be due to chance, statistical bias or effects of confounding factors that are sometimes not evident."[187]
- Boston University epidemiologist Lynn Rosenberg said, "There is evidence that women grossly under-report abortion. . . . An [increase in risk of 30 percent] is indistinguishable from [such bias]. . . . We are certainly not going to arrive at the truth by averaging all the studies."[188]
- American Cancer Society vice president Clark Heath said, "This is a fight between science people and pro-life people. It is a great mistake to start issuing warnings about risks or possible risks when the evidence is so unclear."[189]

The public health establishment attacked small relative risks in this case because liberal abortion rules are sacred among the public health establishment. Small relative risks aren't attacked in the context of secondhand smoke—and indeed, are touted—because smoking is politically incorrect. Get the picture? Weak associations are a dead giveaway of junk science. Size may not matter in other parts of life, but it sure does in epidemiology.

Beware of one trick, though. Junk scientists may try to counter the criticism of a weak association by claiming, "Even a small risk applied to a large population could be a significant public health problem." This is certainly true—but it presumes that relative risk is a measure of risk. It's not.

Relative risk is only a statistical comparison of two study groups. A relative risk may be useful in identifying a statistical difference between the groups that perhaps merits further study. Relative risks do not establish cause-and-effect relationships. Even in the event that an actual cause-and-effect relationship exists, relative risk measures only the difference between two study groups whose members are frequently not randomly selected and not representative of the population.

There's more to evaluating a relative risk than just its size. Next we'll learn how to fight statistics with statistics.

LESSON 6:
BEAT STATISTICS WITH STATISTICS

They drew first blood, not me.

—John Rambo

EPIDEMIOLOGY is statistics. Statistics aren't science. But don't expect a junk scientist to turn to dust when you point that out. You may have to fight statistics with statistics. It's not a scientific argument. But all's fair in love, war—and junk science.

Any given relative risk could have occurred by chance—the same sort of chance that produces heads rather than tails and vice versa. The tool for evaluating the "dumb luck" factor is called "statistical significance." If a relative risk is not statistically significant, you should assume the difference reported between the comparison groups occurred by chance.

The good news is that you don't have to do any work to determine whether a result is statistically significant; the researchers should already have done it for you. If they haven't, then assume the worst—that the relative risk isn't statistically significant. When a relative risk is statistically significant, researchers usually tout it.

You probably will have to obtain a copy of the actual study to check for statistical significance since it rarely is mentioned in media reports. There are two tests for statistical significance of relative risk: the *p*-value and confidence intervals. Don't be intimidated; it's really not complicated.

Rule: 0.05 or Bust

A relative risk indicates whether there is a statistical difference between two study groups being compared. If the relative risk is not exactly 1.0, then some apparent difference between the groups was observed.

But this difference could have occurred by chance. The so-called *p*-value indicates whether the difference occurred by chance. The *p*-value does not evaluate the size of the relative risk, just whether the relative risk is really different from the no-effect level of 1.0.

If the *p*-value indicates the relative risk is not statistically significant, then you can assume that the reported statistical difference between the two study groups occurred by chance and not because there is any true statistical association between the exposure and the disease of interest.

How researchers calculate the *p*-value is not important—whether they calculate it and the result are very important.

Generally speaking, scientists like to be 95 percent sure their results are not due to chance. The 95 percent level is a judgment call, not a law of nature. Nevertheless, it is the traditional level of confidence employed. The *p*-value that corresponds to the 95 percent level of confidence is 0.05. If a *p*-value for a relative risk is 0.05 or less, then the relative risk meets this test of statistical significance.

A recent study reported:

> Compared with nondrinkers, light drinkers who avoided wine had a relative risk for death from all causes of 0.90 . . . and those who drank wine had a relative risk of 0.66. . . . Heavy drinkers who avoided wine were at higher risk for death from all causes than were heavy drinkers who included wine in their alcohol intake. Wine drinkers had signifi-

cantly lower mortality from both coronary heart disease and cancer than did non-wine drinkers ($p = 0.007$ and $p = 0.004$, respectively).[190]

These p-values are much smaller than 0.05, so the observed differences between the groups are deemed unlikely to have occurred by chance. (Of course, this result does not necessarily mean that drinking wine makes you live longer. Remember, the reported relative risks are just statistics and statistics aren't science.)

How can you find out what the p-value is? Look for p-values where relative risks are reported, as in the example above. They will either be labeled as "p-value," or as $p = 0.05$ or whatever the calculated p-value is.

This seems pretty straightforward, but beware of two things. A p-value of 0.05 or less does not transform a statistical association into a causal association. It just means that there is the requisite level of confidence that the observed statistical difference between the comparison groups is not due to chance. Whether the statistical association is in fact a causal association will depend on additional factors.

The p-value is a "killer" test. Though a p-value of 0.05 or less cannot confer "causal" status upon a statistical association, its absence should be regarded as fatal. Many, if not the vast majority of, epidemiologic studies nowadays report relative risks that cannot meet the 0.05 standard. As a consequence, many researchers simply don't report p-values.

If you don't see a p-value reported in a study, it's safe to assume that the relative risk cannot pass this test and the researchers don't want you to know this. The p-value test is such a tough test that, when a relative risk attains the standard, the researcher typically is quite proud to proclaim the p-value.

The p-value test is so feared that some researchers have started a campaign against p-value testing, claiming that it's not a fair way of evaluating epidemiologic results. To be sure, statistical significance testing is not science; it's just statistics. But the p-value test is a traditional statistical tool for evaluating whether statistical results occurred by chance. What the anti-*p*-value campaigners want is a free pass for their junk science. Don't let them have it.

Rule: Just Say No to Intervals Including 1.0

The second part of testing a relative risk for statistical significance is the so-called confidence interval. As with *p*-value testing, researchers traditionally use 95 percent as the standard for confidence intervals.

Remember that a *p*-value tests whether a relative risk different from 1.0 is due to chance. The *p*-value didn't test the size of the relative risk. The confidence interval, though, does. Confidence intervals represent a range of values within which we are 95 percent sure the "true" value of the relative risk lies. Once again, it doesn't matter, for our purposes, how the confidence interval is calculated, only that it is calculated and what its range is.

Positive Association: Lower Bound Greater Than 1.0

For a relative risk greater than 1.0 to satisfy the confidence interval test, the lower value, or "lower bound," of the interval must be greater than 1.0. If the value 1.0 or less is included in the confidence interval, then we cannot be 95 percent sure the true value of the relative risk is greater than 1.0. Here is an example of a relative risk greater than 1.0 that passes the confidence interval test:

> The relative risk of lung cancer was 29.2 (95% CI 5.1, 167.2) for miners with greater than 1,450 working level months compared with those exposed to less than 80 working level months. [Note: The number before the parentheses, 29.2, is the relative risk. The lower and upper bounds of the 95 percent confidence interval (CI) are within the parentheses, 5.1 and 167.2, respectively.][191]

Note that the lower bound of the confidence interval, 5.1, is greater than 1.0.

Here is an example with relative risks greater than 1.0 that *does not* pass the confidence interval test:

> The results . . . suggest [no increase in] specific cancers such as leukemia
> (RR 1.05; CI, 0.82-1.34) and central nervous system tumors (RR 1.04;
> CI, 0.92-1.18).[192]

Note that the lower bounds of the confidence intervals, 0.82 and 0.92, are less than 1.0.

Negative Association: Upper Bound Less Than 1.0

For a relative risk less than 1.0 to satisfy the confidence interval test, the upper bound of the interval must be less than 1.0. If the value 1.0 or greater is included in the confidence interval, then we cannot be 95 percent sure the true value of the relative risk is less than 1.0. Here is an example of relative risks less than 1.0 that pass the confidence interval test:

> Compared with nondrinkers, light drinkers who . . . drank wine had a
> relative risk of 0.66 (CI, 0.55 to 0.77).[193]

Note that the upper bound of the confidence interval, 0.77, is less than 1.0.

Here is an example of relative risks less than 1.0 that *does not* pass the confidence interval test:

> Women reporting the highest level of physical activity at baseline com-
> pared with women with the lowest level of activity had an age-adjusted
> relative risk of breast cancer of 0.92 (95% confidence interval =
> 0.80-1.05).[194]

Note that the upper bound of the confidence interval, 1.05, is greater than 1.0.

As with *p*-value testing, the 95 percent level is not a law of nature. Greater—e.g., 99 percent—or lesser—e.g., 90 percent—values can be used, depending on the confidence desired by the researcher. Here's why different values might be selected.

- A 99 percent confidence interval is wider than a 95 percent confidence interval. Being more confident demands more certainty, which necessitates a greater range of relative risk values.

- A 90 percent confidence interval is narrower than a 95 percent confidence interval. Less confidence requires less certainty, which permits a smaller range of possible relative risk values.

Why do you suppose a junk scientist might want to have a narrower confidence interval?

Moving the Statistical Goalposts

What if the lower bound of a 95 percent confidence interval was less than 1.0? Then the results would not be statistically significant. But suppose a 90 percent confidence interval narrowed the confidence interval, pulling the lower bound up to about 1.0. The result would be statistically significant. That's a trick used by the U.S. Environmental Protection Agency in its infamous study on secondhand smoke and lung cancer. The judge in that case wrote:

> Plaintiffs raise a list of objections asserting that EPA deviated from accepted scientific procedure and its own Risk Assessment Guidelines in a manner designed to ensure a preordained outcome. Given the ETS Risk Assessment shortcomings already discussed, it is neither necessary or desirable to delve further into EPA's epidemiological web. However, two of Plaintiffs' arguments require mention. The first contention is EPA switched, without explanation, from using standard 95% confidence intervals to 90% confidence intervals to enhance the likelihood that its meta-analysis would appear statistically significant. This shift assisted EPA in obtaining statistically significant results. Studies that are not statistically significant are "null studies"; they cannot support a Group A classification. See Brock v. Merrell Dow Pharm., Inc., 874 F.2d 307, 312 (5th Cir. 1989) ("If the confidence interval is so great that it includes the number 1.0, then the study will be said to show no statistically significant association between the factor and the disease.").
>
> EPA used a 95% confidence interval in the 1990 Draft ETS Risk Assessment, but later switched to a 90% confidence interval. Most prominently, this drew criticism from . . . a contributor to the ETS Risk Assessment: "The use of 90% confidence intervals, instead of the conventionally used 95% confidence intervals, is to be discouraged. It looks like a[n] attempt to achieve statistical significance for a result which otherwise would not achieve significance."

The record and EPA's explanations to the court make it clear that using standard methodology, EPA could not produce statistically significant results with its selected studies. Analysis conducted with a .05 significance level and 95% confidence level included relative risks of 1. Accordingly, these results did not confirm EPA's controversial a priori hypothesis. In order to confirm its hypothesis, EPA maintained its standard significant level but lowered the confidence interval to 90%. This allowed EPA to confirm its hypothesis by finding a relative risk of 1.19, albeit a very weak association.[195]

Ninety-five percent is the standard value for epidemiologic research. Beware of those who try to skirt this standard.

There's one more thing to consider about confidence intervals. The confidence interval indicates the range of likely values of the relative risk. A "too-wide" confidence interval is not good; it is an indication that the underlying data are unusually disparate, including "outliers" and oddball data values. A "tight" confidence interval indicates more uniformity, less variance among the data. Consider the following example:

The relative risk of lung cancer was 29.2 (95% CI 5.1, 167.2) for miners [who worked for more than 8.5 months in uranium mines] compared with those [who worked for less than two weeks in uranium mines].[196]

In this case, the "true" relative risk may be 5 times larger (167.2) than the reported relative risk (29.2). It may also be one-sixth the size of the estimated relative risk. So the relative risk is subject to great fluctuation. This is not good. It's much better to have a tighter confidence interval, like this:

Compared with nondrinkers, light drinkers who . . . drank wine had a relative risk of [death of] 0.66 (CI, 0.55 to 0.77).[197]

The reported reduction in relative risk of death among wine drinkers is 0.34 (1.0 minus 0.66). The upper and lower confidence intervals are only 0.11—or one-third the size of the reported effect (0.34)—higher and lower, respectively, than the estimate of relative risk (0.66). Compare this with the prior example where the upper and lower bounds were more than five times greater and less than the size of the effect.

When is a confidence interval "too wide"? When is it sufficiently "tight"? Unfortunately, there are no rules—although I tend to doubt relative risks where the confidence interval is larger than the reported size of the observed effect—i.e., a potential 100 percent variation in the relative risk isn't a confidence builder.

LESSON 7:
BIG NUMBERS MEAN BIG LIES

There are two kinds of statistics,
the kind you look up, and the kind you make up.

—Rex Stout

"BODY COUNTS" are a great way to grab the public's attention. The bigger, the better. Smoking kills 400,000 per year. Obesity kills 300,000 per year. Drug reactions kill 100,000 per year. Medical mistakes kill 98,000 per year. Secondhand smoke kills 50,000 per year. Radon kills 10,000 per year.

Body counts, or rather "noncounts," are simply more statistical malpractice. Let's see if you can figure out why.

Beware: Relative Risk Ahead

Epidemiologists estimate body counts by using the formula for "attributable fraction" (AF):

$$AF = \frac{\text{Proportion of population with characteristic x (relative risk} - 1)}{\text{Proportion of population with characteristic x (relative risk} - 1) + 1} \times 100\%$$

Without even understanding the formula or actually working through an example, you should already see what the problem is—reliance on relative risk. (See Lesson 4: Epidemiology Is Statistics.) The attributable risk formula pretends that relative risk indicates risk.

As we know, relative risks can be used only for statistically associating an exposure with a disease. The greater the relative risk, the more confident we may be that there is a real statistical association between exposure and disease. But relative risk does not prove that a cause-and-effect association exists. The attributable fraction formula simply ignores this inconvenient fact. Consider this quasi-hypothetical example.

Let's say that 20 percent of the U.S. population lives in areas where the level of fine particulate air pollution exceeds a level statistically associated with a 17 percent increase in death rates from cardiopulmonary diseases. The question for the junk scientist, then, is how many deaths will be caused by the fine particulate air pollution? Plugging the numbers into our attributable fraction formula, we have

$$\text{AF of cardiopulmonary deaths from air pollution} = \frac{.20 \times (1.17 - 1)}{.20 \times (1.17 - 1) + 1}$$
$$= \frac{0.034}{1.034}$$
$$= 3.3 \text{ percent}$$

The junk scientist would conclude that 3.3 percent of all cardiopulmonary deaths are caused by fine particulate air pollution. So, if there are 1 million deaths in the United States annually from cardiopulmonary causes, then 3.3. percent of these—or 33,000—are caused by fine particulate air pollution.

The fatal defect in this junk science exercise is the assumption that the relative risk really means that fine particulate air pollution increases death rates by 17 percent. We've already discussed how the study reporting the relative risk of 1.17 was ecologic in nature. It merely statistically associated death rates with air pollution levels on a geographic basis. No one knows how much air pollution any of the deceased subjects were exposed to, and no one made clinical evaluations establishing fine particulate matter as the cause of the observed deaths.

Attributable fraction and attributable risk—the number derived by applying the attributable fraction to the number of deaths—is statistical abuse squared.

Here's what the editors of the *New England Journal of Medicine* had to say about the estimate that obesity kills 300,000 per year:

> Unfortunately, the data linking overweight and death, as well as the data showing the beneficial effects of weight loss, are limited, fragmentary, and often ambiguous. Most of the evidence is either indirect or derived from observational epidemiologic studies, many of which have serious methodologic flaws. Many studies fail to consider confounding variables, which are extremely difficult to assess and control for in this type of study. For example, mortality among obese people may be misleadingly high because overweight people are more likely to be sedentary and of low socioeconomic status. Thus, although some claim that every year 300,000 deaths in the United States are caused by obesity, that figure is by no means well established. Not only is it derived from weak or incomplete data, but it is also called into question by the methodologic difficulties of determining which of many factors contribute to premature death [references omitted].[198]

In response to a flurry of letters from the junk science mob, the editors further stated:

> Calculations of attributable risk are fraught with problems. They provide only an upper bound for the effect of a single variable, because many other factors, both recognized and unrecognized, may also be contributing to the outcome. When several known factors are taken into account, it is even possible to find that they account for more than 100 percent of deaths—a nonsensical result.[199]

And here you have it: Body noncounts = Attributable risk = "Nonsensical."

Junk Science Economics

An up-and-coming tactic among the junk science mob is putting price tags on "bad behavior." Smoking costs society $72 billion per year in health care costs. Alcohol abuse costs $250 billion per year. Obesity costs $40 billion. These "price tags" have faults corresponding to those of "body counts."

Study: California Spends $8.7 Billion
for Smoking-Related Health Care

was the Associated Press headline for September 9, 1998. The article continued,

> Counting all sources of medical payments, the total cost of caring for people with cigarette-related health care problems is estimated at $72.7 billion a year, almost six times the $12.9 billion estimated cost to Medicaid alone, according to a study published Wednesday in Public Health Reports.

But there was much more to this news than the AP reported. The reported dollar figures were based on a statistic called the "smoking attributable fraction" (SAF). The researchers described the SAF as follows:

> To estimate SAFs, we [estimated] the expected expenditures for medical care of smokers and the expected expenditures for medical care of a hypothetical group of [never-smokers]. The difference in expected expenditures between the two groups is allocatable to smoking. The ratio of the expenditures allocatable to smoking to total expenditures is the fraction of expenditures attributable to smoking, the SAF.[200]

So the dollar figures are based on the assumption that differences in medical expenditures between smokers and nonsmokers are due only to smoking. This is probably not true.

Smokers tend to have a panoply of "unhealthy" habits, including not exercising, poorer diet, higher alcohol consumption, more stress, being less health conscious, and being of lower socioeconomic status. Much of the difference in medical expenditures between smokers and nonsmokers could be due to these lifestyle differences as well as to smoking.

When you read or hear about these big numbers, laugh out loud. I do.

LESSON 8:
BOYCOTT BIOASSAYS

I didn't think; I experimented.
—Wilhelm Roentgen

JUNK SCIENTISTS OFTEN try to scare you with the results of experiments called "bioassays," in which chemicals are tested on laboratory animals, usually mice or rats. While there certainly may be merit in testing chemicals on laboratory animals, the bioassay technique is often abused.

Rule: Mice Aren't Little People

Scientists reported in the early 1970s that saccharin caused bladder cancer in rats. This led to calls for banning saccharin. But the finding was controversial. It was, after all, based on a study of rats. Studies of human populations didn't report persuasive evidence of increased cancer rates among saccharin users, even though saccharin had been on the market for decades. Although saccharin wasn't banned from human consumption, products containing it had to be labeled to the effect that saccharin caused cancer in laboratory animals.

A quarter century after the rats got cancer, the World Health Organization's International Agency for Research on Cancer (IARC) let saccharin off the hook in 1999:

> Sodium saccharin produces urothelial bladder tumours in rats by a non-DNA-reactive mechanism that involves the formation of a urinary calcium phosphate-containing precipitate, cytotoxicity and enhanced cell proliferation. This mechanism is *not relevant* to humans because of critical interspecies differences in urine composition. (Emphasis added)[201]

So saccharin causes bladder tumors in rats through a biological process that humans simply don't have. As you might have expected, the rats weren't little people.

Government Underestimates Infant Exposure to Toxic Weed Killer

was the title of the July 1999 media release touting "Into the Mouths of Babes," a report by an environmental activist group.[202] The release began,

> The toxic weed killer atrazine is polluting tap water in almost 800 Midwestern communities, and the government has underestimated exposure to the carcinogen by 15 times for infants fed formula mixed with tap water. . . .

Is atrazine a carcinogen?

IARC concluded, "There is sufficient evidence in experimental animals for the carcinogenicity of atrazine."[203] But IARC also noted:

> There are critical interspecies differences in the hormonal changes associated with reproductive senescence. Therefore, there is strong evidence that the mechanism by which atrazine increases the incidence of mammary gland tumours in Sprague-Dawley rats is not relevant to humans.

Oops.

Another example of critical biological differences between laboratory animals and humans involves unleaded gasoline. In 1991, the U.S. Environmental Protection Agency decided not to classify unleaded gasoline as cancer causing despite evidence that unleaded gasoline increased cancer rates in two species of animals—kidney tumors in male rats and liver tumors in female mice.[204]

Typically, evidence of cancer-causing potential in both sexes of two species is sufficient for classifying a substance as a carcinogen. But the EPA decided that the evidence for unleaded gasoline's increasing kidney tumor rates in male mice wasn't relevant to humans. The kidney tumors in the rats were caused by the accumulation of a certain protein. That protein is present in male rats, not in female rats and, more significant, not in humans.

Mice and people both are mammals and have much biology in common. But mice and people differ in many obvious—and not so obvious—ways. These differences make it unwise to assume that chemicals act the same in laboratory rodents and people.

Rule: Humans Aren't Cancer Time Bombs
Chemical testing is generally conducted in the animal species thought to be the most likely to show an adverse health effect—"most sensitive species" testing. The animals typically are bred to have a higher rate of spontaneously developed cancer.

Cancer Time Bombs
Sprague-Dawley rats, Fischer (F-344) rats, and B6C3F1 mice are cancer time bombs. As was pointed out by Phil Abelson, editor emeritus of *Science:*

> The use of inbred strains as test animals can further be questioned on the basis that they often develop spontaneous tumors in organs where cancers are not frequent in humans. For example, incidences of mouse liver tumors in 2-year-old B6C3F1 males have ranged from 17.8 to 46.9 percent. In contrast, death rate from liver cancer in the United States is about 0.005 percent.[205]

And that's not all. The inbreeding of these animals may also cause other problems. Abelson editorialized in *Science:*

> Most standard risk assessment experiments expose rodents to large doses of a test chemical for about 2 years, which is approximately their natural life-span. For most tests, one or more of three strains of rodents are

used: Sprague-Dawley (SD) rats, Fischer (F-344) rats, and B6C3F1 mice. These animals have a higher natural incidence of tumors than do humans, and some of the tumors are not common to humans. These rodent strains were adopted in the belief that they would exhibit less variability than wild-type animals do. On the basis of this assumption, enormous effort has been expended in studies of about 500 different chemicals. Each experiment has involved comparison between dosed and nondosed animals (controls). Thus a large database is available concerning the weight, longevity, and pathology of control animals. Data cited in the Toxicology Forum proceedings and in Dietary Restriction indicate that, during the past 25 to 30 years, the adult body weight of rodents from most of the strains used in toxicity testing has increased 20 to 30%. Degenerative diseases and tumor incidence also have increased. Rodent survival has decreased. At the Merck Research Laboratory in the 1970s, the survival rate at age 2 of SD rats used as controls was 58%. In the 1980s it was 44%, and in the 1990s it had dropped to 24%. A different laboratory compiled data on F-344 rats. In 1970, 80% of males survived for 2 years. In 1981, 60% survived. Their current survival rate is 36%. The incidence of tumors in control rodents has also changed with time. For example, the number of liver tumors in control B6C3F1 mice increased from an average of 32% in 1980 to about 50% in 1984. In tests at various laboratories, liver tumor incidence in male B6C3F1 mice has varied between 10 and 76%.

A partial explanation for this variability in longevity and health lies in practices at the breeder companies. Apparently, they have unwittingly caused genetic drift by their methods of selecting breeding stock. The standardized procedure at risk assessment laboratories has also been a factor. In general, animals are fed ad libitum (ad lib); that is, they are given as much food as they want to eat. As a result of overeating, the health of ad lib animals is impaired. This is clearly shown by the fact that if the food intake of littermates of ad lib animals is reduced to 70% or less of ad lib amounts, rodent health and longevity are much improved. A recent experiment using SD rats compared the longevity of control rats fed ad lib with that of rats fed 65% of the ad lib amounts. At maturity, the ad lib males weighed 60% more than did the diet-restricted males. Only 7% of the ad lib males lived as long as 2 years. In contrast, 72% of the diet-restricted rats survived for more than 2 years. They were sleek and healthy. Although this phenomenon has been widely observed and well known for many years, the standard protocol still calls for ad lib feeding, so that in effect, when animals are exposed to chemicals in risk assessments, they simultaneously receive one potential carcinogen and one known carcinogen—their food.[206]

You know there's a problem when food is a cancer-causing substance.

Not only are mice not people, in many respects laboratory mice aren't even mice anymore. And if you think that pretending that mice are little people is kind of weird, wait until you see what gets done to the mice.

Science or Divination?

Haruspicy is the ancient practice of predicting the future by examining the livers and entrails of sacrificed animals. Bioassays are a modern analog.

Although haruspicy is commonly believed to be of Etruscan origin (the advanced civilization in Italy before the rise of Rome about 3,000 years ago), the ancient Sumerians also foretold the future by reading animal entrails. The Sumerians, though, were smart enough not to write down their predictions. Our society, on the other hand, turns haruspicy-based predictions into law.

Polychlorinated biphenyls (PCBs) are chemicals once widely used as hydraulic and insulating fluids. Researcher Renate D. Kimbrough et al. reported in 1975 the results of feeding rats high doses of a PCB:

> Sherman strain female rats (200) were fed 100 [parts per million] of [a PCB] for approximately 21 months, and 200 female rats were kept as controls. The rats were killed when 23 months old. Twenty-six of 184 experimental animals and 1 of 173 controls had liver cancer. None of the controls but 146 of 184 experimental rats had [abnormal] nodules in their livers, and areas of [liver cell] alteration were noted in 28 of 173 controls and 182 of 184 experimental animals. Thus the [PCB], when fed in the diet, had a [cancer-causing] effect in these rats. The incidence of tumors in other organs did not differ appreciably between the experimental and control groups.[207]

The ensuing panic helped passage of a new federal law banning the manufacture of PCBs in 1976. President Jimmy Carter said about the new law, "Rather than coping with [hazards such as PCBs] after they have escaped into our environment, our primary objective must be to prevent them from entering the environment at all."[208]

At the time, it was believed that anywhere from 60 to 90 percent of cancers could be caused by exposure to environmental contaminants. President Carter favored increased emphasis on preventing cancer rather than searching for elusive cancer cures. The problem, though, was that no study at the time linked PCBs with increased cancer risk in humans. Little has changed. In fact, it was Dr. Kimbrough who demonstrated the folly of predicting human cancer risk from laboratory animal experiments.

In March 1999, Kimbrough published the results of the largest-ever study of workers who had been highly exposed to PCBs:[209] No increase in cancer deaths was reported among the workers—not even among the most highly exposed workers. Oh, well. Another law without a scientific basis.

Bioassays may seem like a sensible approach to testing chemicals for cancer-causing potential—and perhaps they were 25 years ago when little was known about chemical exposures and cancer. While laboratory animal testing may often provide useful information on the potential toxicity of a chemical, high-dose experiments used to predict human cancer risk are pure folly.

Here are the rules for evaluating laboratory animal experiments—should you bother to consider animal testing at all.

Rule: Real Cancer Risks Occur in Real People

Remember the phenolphthalein that Schering-Plough advertised *wasn't* in its products? Researchers fed genetically engineered mice many times the amount of phenolphthalein that a human would actually use. When higher cancer rates were observed in the mice, the FDA jumped to the conclusion that phenolphthalein posed a cancer risk to humans.

The FDA ignored that phenolphthalein had been used as an ingredient in laxatives for more than 100 years—with no indication of human cancer-causing potential. Epidemiologic studies so far have failed even to statistically associate laxatives with increased rates of cancer.[210] The available data show only that the FDA should stop poisoning mice with phenolphthalein. Before believing the results of a bioassay, check out the available data on humans.

Rule: Poisoning Animals Is Probability, Not Science

Bioassays typically involve plying animals with mega-doses of chemicals. The rationale is probability, not science. Researchers count on high doses maximizing the chances of observing toxic effects. But how relevant are high doses to actual human exposures?

Remember the Alar scare? Even assuming that Alar increased cancer risk at the doses tested in mice, a human would have to drink 19,000 quarts of apple juice every day for life to consume an amount of Alar proportionate to that fed the mice.

Dioxin Can Harm Tooth Development

headlined *Science News* on February 20, 1999. The article continued:

> In the early 1980s, a Finnish dentist noticed that an unusually large share of her young patients had soft, discolored molars. Because the affected teeth had emerged bearing structural defects, she suspected that during infancy, when the teeth were forming beneath the gums, the children had been exposed to some toxic compound. The culprit now appears to be breast milk tainted with dioxins, says Satu Alaluusua of the University of Helsinki Institute of Dentistry. . . . To probe whether the defects that she was observing might reflect a more moderate exposure to the same pollutants, Alaluusua began exposing adult rats to . . . the most potent dioxin. "We saw a similar mottling of teeth," as well as malformations in their mineral structure, she told Science News.[211]

What Alaluusua didn't tell *Science News*—or at least what *Science News* didn't report—was that the dose of dioxin given the rats was 1,000 micrograms per kilogram of body weight—a near lethal amount for rats and millions of times more dioxin than humans are exposed to.[212]

Maximizing the chances of observing a toxic effect means minimizing the chances a bioassay has any relevance to humans.

Rule: Poisoning May Be Toxic

Birth defects among the offspring of treated animals in a bioassay aren't necessarily caused by the substance being tested. The birth defects could be a secondary effect, caused by the treated mothers being sickened while pregnant. Remember, the mothers are typically given very high doses of the substance.

The "food police" at the Center for Science in the Public Interest started a jihad against caffeine in 1976. CSPI urged the federal government to warn pregnant women to lower their caffeine consumption on the basis of studies reporting birth defects among the offspring of female mice fed high doses of caffeine.[213]

The CSPI petitioned the U.S. Food and Drug Administration in November 1979 to label coffee and tea for caffeine content and, once again, issue warnings to pregnant women.[214] CSPI suggested that removing caffeine from cola drinks was another option. In March 1980, CSPI held a press conference to announce the Caffeine Birth Defects Clearinghouse.

The FDA soon caved, issuing a September 1980 warning to pregnant women to minimize their consumption of coffee, tea, and colas—even though, the FDA acknowledged, the evidence wasn't conclusive.[215] But this wasn't enough for CSPI, which continued to insist that the animal test results justified warning labels. What were these results? Baby rats had been born with missing parts of toes when their mothers were force fed caffeine at the human equivalent of 24 cups of coffee per day.[216]

The CSPI's campaign unraveled soon enough, though. In June 1981, a review panel at the National Institute of Environmental Health Sciences concluded that the pregnant rats may simply have been poisoned by the high doses of caffeine. This caused them to lose weight and the weight loss itself affected the development of the baby rats.

Still, the FDA still maintains its 1980 warning to pregnant women. CSPI still insists, "Knowing the caffeine content is important to many people—especially women who are or might become pregnant."[217]

The Bottom Line on Animal Testing

The U.S. government's National Toxicology Program relies on bioassays to test and classify chemicals for their potential to cause cancer. Researchers recently estimated that 85 percent of the chemicals tested in the NTP's bioassays were either carcinogenic or anti-carcinogenic at some site in some sex-species group. The authors concluded, "This suggests that most chemicals given at high enough doses will cause some sort of perturbation in tumor rates."[218]

Does this mean perhaps that basing public policy and health scares on poisoned animals isn't such a good idea after all? Should the NTP be renamed "Not Too Probative"? Are bioassays bioassinine?

LESSON 9:
EXPOSURE ISN'T TOXICITY

*All substances are poisons, there is none which is
not a poison.
The right dose differentiates a poison and a remedy.*

—Paracelsus

A REALITY OF MODERN life is regular contact with a variety of manmade—and Mother Nature's—chemicals. Chemicals are in the air we breathe, the food we eat, the water we drink, and the consumer products we use. Exposure to manmade chemicals is unavoidable, no matter what you do or where you go.

No Harm, No Foul

The good news is that no observable harm is caused by the vast majority of exposures to chemicals. Short of poisoning, chemical exposures are essentially harmless. The bad news is that the Junksters don't want you to know that. They want you to believe that your health is in jeopardy unless you live in a pristine environment, consume "natural" or "organic" products, and avoid all exposure to manmade chemicals.

The most common ploy is an attempt to scare the public with a new study reporting that a manmade chemical has been "discovered" in humans or in the air, water, or food. A classic example is the February 8, 1990, media release from the North Carolina Department of Agriculture that blared

Benzene Found in Perrier
Water Health Warning Issued

Benzene was measured in samples of Perrier at levels of about 15 parts per billion, exceeding U.S. public drinking water standards set at 5 parts per billion.

But remember that regulatory levels are set way below "safe" levels. The levels of benzene found in Perrier were not and are not known to cause any health effects whatsoever. Regulators merely *assumed* that, because *long-term*, *ultra-high* exposures to benzene *may* have caused health effects in *some* people, any exposure is harmful.

Rule: The Dose Makes the Poison

Sixteenth-century physician Paracelsus observed that specific chemicals cause the toxic effects of plant and animal poisons. He documented that human response to those chemicals depended on the dose received, revealing that small doses of a substance might be harmless or even beneficial whereas larger doses could be toxic.

Using these observations, Paracelsus developed a treatment for syphilis that used mercury, a substance that is toxic to humans at a sufficiently high dose. At lower doses, though, mercury apparently had a therapeutic effect. Paracelsus' treatment was used for more than 350 years until German bacteriologist Paul Ehrlich developed a treatment using arsenic (also a poison at higher doses).

It is a fundamental principle of toxicology that "the dose makes the poison." Two or three aspirin will cure your headache. Two hundred will kill you. There is even a lethal dose of water. The corresponding junk science principle is "any dose is poison." The Junksters count on your not knowing that exposure isn't toxicity.

Rule: Use Does Not Equal Exposure

The implication that exposure equals toxicity is often accompanied by the equally dubious implication that "use of a chemical means exposure to the chemical." The combination of these implications is "use equals toxicity." Don't fall for it.

Breast Cancer Study Flags Lawn Pesticides

blazoned *USA Today* on October 21, 1999. The article continued:

> Researchers seeking clues about the high rate of breast cancer among wealthy women have found potential environmental factors, including professional lawn and dry-cleaning services.
>
> Focusing on the Boston suburb of Newton, the researchers found women in areas hit hardest by the disease used such services more often than those in less-affected neighborhoods. The study showed that women in neighborhoods with higher rates of breast cancer typically had higher incomes and education levels than women in areas with lower breast cancer rates. . . . But the survey did suggest possible environmental factors. For example, 65% of the women in the area with higher breast-cancer rates had used a professional lawn service, compared with 36% of the women in the low-incidence neighborhood.
>
> In addition, 30% of those in the high-incidence area reported routine use of pesticides, compared with 23% in the low-incidence sector. And 45% of those in the high-incidence area used dry cleaning at least once a month, compared with 32% in the less-affected neighborhood.

This report tries to equate mere use of pesticides and dry-cleaning services—not actual exposure to the chemicals—with breast cancer. No data were collected on the women's exposures, if any, to the chemicals.

"Use" of chemicals does not equate to exposure to them, much less dangerous exposure. If pesticides are used according to the directions, exposure is minimized if not eliminated. Exposure to pesticides is even less likely if a lawn service is employed.

Wealthy white women typically have higher rates of breast cancer than black, Hispanic, poor, and rural women.[219] It's no surprise that wealth correlates with pesticide, lawn service, and dry-cleaning use—wealthier individuals are more likely to use and can more easily afford those products and services. Higher rates of breast cancer also probably correlate with purchasing organic foods and driving Volvo station wagons.

A fundamental tenet of toxicology—the study of poisons—is that "the dose makes the poison." That is, every substance is toxic at a sufficiently high level of exposure. The corollary is that a substance is not toxic at sufficiently low levels of exposure. Consequently, exposure does not equal toxicity.

Rule: There's Always a "Safe" Exposure

Junksters like to alarm the public by saying that there are no safe levels of exposure to cancer-causing substances. This alarmism has even been enshrined in law and regulation. Under the Safe Drinking Water Act, for example, the U.S. Environmental Protection Agency establishes goals of zero exposure for drinking water contaminants associated with cancer.

One such substance is dioxin, a ubiquitous byproduct of many industrial processes (e.g., chemical manufacturing and incineration), consumer activities (e.g., automobile tailpipe exhaust and fireplace wood burning), and natural processes (forest fires and volcanic eruptions).

Over the past 25 years, environmental activists have portrayed dioxin as "the most toxic substance known to man." Dioxin was the contaminant of concern at the infamous Love Canal and Times Beach environmental "disasters" and in the Vietnam-era defoliant Agent Orange.

The EPA has been "reassessing" the alleged hazards of dioxin for almost 10 years. The agency's 1994 effort to label dioxin as a "known human carcinogen" was rejected by its board of independent science advisers. Back from the drawing board in June 2000, the EPA urged that dioxin be labeled an even more potent human carcinogen.

Environmental activists extrapolating from the EPA's report claimed that 1 of every 14 cancers is caused by the dioxin in our bodies and from unavoidable daily exposures through food and the environment.[220] Allegedly, dioxin causes a variety of developmental, behavioral, and immune problems in children.

Following the EPA's announcement of its tentative conclusions, the environmental activist group Center for Health, Environment and Justice placed a full-page advertisement in the *New York Times* picturing a breakfast and pointing to all the foods containing dioxin, including an omelet's eggs and cheese, bacon, sausage, cream, milk, and butter. The ad states that dioxin is "the most toxic man-made substance on earth. . . . And you had some for breakfast. And you'll have some for lunch. And for dinner. . . ." Scary stuff. What's a consumer to do? That's where Ben & Jerry's ice cream comes to the rescue.

As I enjoyed some Ben & Jerry's ice cream at one of its "scoop shops" during the summer of 1999, I noticed a Ben & Jerry's marketing brochure titled "Our Thoughts on Dioxin." The brochure stated, "Dioxin is known to cause cancer, genetic and reproductive defects and learning disabilities. . . . The only safe level of dioxin exposure is no exposure at all."

Knowing that dioxin is in virtually all food, Dr. Michael Gough and I put Ben & Jerry's ice cream to the test. Gough is a former government scientist who chaired the U.S. Department of Health and Human Services advisory panel on the effects of dioxin-contaminated Agent Orange on U.S. Air Force personnel in Vietnam and served as one of EPA's science advisers in the 1994 review of dioxin.

We measured the level of dioxin in a sample of Ben & Jerry's World's Best Vanilla ice cream. We presented the results at the Dioxin 2000 scientific conference held in Monterey, California.[221]

Two independent laboratories using different methodologies reported that a single serving of the ice cream contained about 200 times the level of dioxin the EPA says is "safe"—according to the existing EPA standard. Under the EPA's new estimate of the cancer risk from dioxin—10 times higher than the old one—a serving of Ben & Jerry's would exceed the safe level by a whopping 2,000 times. The level would be about 7,400 times what the EPA says is safe for a 40-pound child.

If dioxin is so dangerous—as Ben & Jerry's and Greenpeace, the ice cream maker's science adviser, seem to think it is—then how can Ben & Jerry's sell its ice cream? Doesn't the company care about the children?—a segment of the population continually exploited to promote the political and social agendas of the EPA and environmental activists.

The answer, of course, is that the low levels of dioxin in our food and the environment are not dangerous. There are "safe" levels of exposure to dioxin. And if dioxin is the most toxic manmade substance, then there are "safe" exposures to all other manmade chemicals, too.

LESSON 10:
MIND THE MYTHS

He that knows little often repeats it.

— Anonymous

MANY HEALTH SCARES are ingrained in our culture. They've been pounded into our heads thanks to endless repetition by mindless media. Junk science–based myths may serve as rationales for new health scares, so it pays to beware of them.

You'll run into these health scare myths regularly. Don't be bamboozled. Here are some biggies.

Myth: Agent Orange Causes Cancer

Some epidemiologic studies report statistical associations between exposure to herbicides contaminated with dioxins and cancer. Agent Orange, used during the Vietnam War, is one such herbicide.

Some Vietnam veterans' groups latched onto these studies and bullied the U.S. government into compensating them for a variety of diseases, including cancer. But no scientific study of Vietnam veterans credibly links exposure to Agent Orange with cancer risk, including these:

- In a study of 329 Vietnam-era veterans with a diagnosis of lung cancer made between 1983 and 1990, researchers wrote, "We conclude from these data that there is no evidence of increased risk in lung cancer associated with service in Vietnam at this time."[222]
- Rearchers studied 87 Vietnamese women with gestational trophoblastic disease (i.e., hydatidiform mole and choriocarcinoma) and reported, "No significant difference [in disease rate] was found between cases and controls for this index (OR = 0.7, 95% CI = 0.2-1.8 for high-exposure category), nor was such a difference noted for the agricultural use of pesticides."[223]
- Researchers studied 283 Vietnam-era veterans and reported, "Surrogate measures of potential Agent Orange exposure such as service in a specific military branch, in a certain region within Vietnam, in a combat role, or extended Vietnam service time were not associated with any significant increased risk of Hodgkin's Disease."[224]
- Researchers studied 201 Vietnam-era veterans and concluded: "Service in Vietnam did not increase the risk of non-Hodgkin's lymphoma either in general (branch adjusted odds ratio = 1.03, 95% confidence interval = 0.70-1.50) or with increased latency period as defined as the duration in years from first service in Vietnam to hospital discharge. Surrogate measures of potential Agent Orange exposure such as service in a specific military branch, in a certain region within Vietnam, or in a combat role as determined by military occupational speciality were not associated with any increased risk of non-Hodgkin's lymphoma."[225]
- Researchers studied 568 Vietnam veterans with a variety of cancers and concluded, "These results provide no evidence that, 15 to 25 years following service in Vietnam, the risk of these malignant neoplasms is higher among veterans."[226]

- Researchers studying 995 U.S. Air Force veterans of Operation Ranch Hand, the unit responsible for aerial spraying of herbicides in Vietnam, reported no increase in melanoma and systemic cancers.[227]

Though study of health effects among Vietnam veterans potentially caused by Agent Orange continues, there's no evidence of a link with cancer—even a statistical one.

Myth: Pollution Causes Cancer Clusters

Remember the movie *A Civil Action*? John Travolta starred as a personal injury lawyer crusading for "justice"—unabashedly in the form of millions of dollars—against two companies accused of dumping chemicals in Woburn, Massachusetts, during the 1970s. Allegedly, the chemicals contaminated drinking water, causing eight children's deaths from leukemia—four times the "average" rate. This geographic grouping of the children's cancer is called a "cancer cluster."

The movie recounted the lawsuit filed against W. R. Grace and Beatrice Foods in the 1980s. The jury vindicated Beatrice Foods. W. R. Grace settled for $8 million, disappointing the plaintiff's attorneys who couldn't prove the company illegally dumped chemicals. The movie pretty much ended there, anti-climactically, except for the final legend:

> In 1996, fifteen years after Jimmy Anderson's death, the Massachusetts Dept. of Health made an official finding that the contaminants in the water were indeed responsible for causing the leukemia in the children.

The legend was true enough. The Massachusetts Department of Health did make such a finding. But you shouldn't be surprised to learn that such an "official" finding is a far cry from a "scientific" one.

Science has yet to demonstrate that the cancer cluster of the Woburn tragedy had anything to do with chemicals, notwithstanding the Massachusetts Department of Health. The most timely investigation of the Woburn cancer cluster, which included interviews with Woburn residents, reported that (1) the victims weren't different from leukemia-free neighbors, (2) the contaminants at issue aren't known to cause leukemia, and (3) no victim had contact with the hazardous waste sites in question.

The Massachusetts Department of Health declaration, in contrast, is based on a 20-years-after-the-fact guess of what could possibly have happened. Such revisionism hardly constitutes "science."

Can the Woburn cancer cluster be explained? It's likely the tragedy is simply a chance occurrence. Just by chance, some areas have higher rates of cancer than others. Reports of cancer "clusters" rarely—if ever—have any other explanation.

Don't take my word for it, though. Here's a report from the Centers for Disease Control and Prevention:

> Beginning in 1961, the Centers for Disease Control investigated 108 cancer clusters and reported the findings in Epidemic Aid Reports. The clusters studied were of leukemia (38%), leukemia and lymphoma (30%), leukemia and other cancer combinations (13%), and all other cancer or combinations (19%). These clusters occurred in 29 states and five foreign countries, with the largest numbers from Connecticut (11), California (eight), Illinois (eight), New York (eight), Georgia (seven), Pennsylvania (six), and Iowa (five). All other states reported less than five. Eight different data collection methods were used, often in combinations, and four types of laboratory methods on four different specimen types. Although 14 different categories of associations were reported, no clear cause was found for any cluster.[228]

Cancer cluster investigations have been such a bust that public health officials have developed public-response strategies to avoid what are considered little more than wild goose chases.

Minnesota, which investigated more than 1,000 cancer clusters from 1984 to 1995, hasn't conducted a formal investigation in several years. "The reality is that [cancer cluster investigations] are an absolute, total and complete waste of taxpayer dollars," says Alan Bender, a Minnesota state epidemiologist.[229] And researchers recently reported:

> A mail survey was sent to state health departments requesting data [on requests for cancer cluster investigations] for 1997. Approximately 1100

cluster investigation requests were made in 1997. Most requests were made by citizens, and no pattern emerged for types of cancer or hazards suspected. States rate this work as average in importance and feel satisfied with the [success] of their communication efforts. Few cluster inquiries require further investigation.[230]

Why do cancer cluster investigations amount to wild goose chases?

Statistically significant clusters can occur by chance.[231] Any search for biologically meaningful causes will be severely constrained by various methodologic difficulties, including long and probably variable latent periods between causative events and cancer diagnosis, the limited numbers of cases available for study in any given cluster situation, and the clinical nonspecificity of cancer cases, which means no readily available tools are at hand for identifying the specific causes for any particular case.[232]

So when you hear about a cancer cluster, treat it the way your local public health department would—don't waste your time.

Myth: Chernobyl Caused Thousands of Fatal Cancers

"A nuclear power critic said . . . the Chernobyl accident will cause 1 million cancer cases worldwide, half of them fatal—an estimate sharply higher than those made by other experts," reported the Associated Press in the aftermath of the nuclear accident at Chernobyl.[233] The article continued:

> Dr. John Gofman, a medical physicist at the University of California in Berkeley, presented his conclusions about the Soviet Union's April 26 accident during an American Chemical Society meeting.
> "Dr. Gofman has a history of exaggerating risk estimates for radiation," said Dr. Arthur Upton, a former director of the National Cancer Institute. Upton expects 5,000 to 10,000 Chernobyl-linked cancer deaths.

Gofman was wrong. And so far, Upton too. The BBC reported on June 13, 2000:

The Chernobyl nuclear disaster had less impact on public health than was initially feared, according to UN data cited by the International Atomic Energy Agency (IAEA).

About 1,800 children did develop thyroid cancer, a treatable disease which is rarely fatal, and more cases are expected, an IAEA statement said on Tuesday.

"However, with this exception, there is no scientific evidence of increases in overall cancer incidence or mortality or in non-malignant disorders that could be related to radiation exposure," it said.

Thirty-one people died from radiation poisoning in the explosion and its immediate aftermath. Health experts feared that thousands living nearby would develop cancers as a result of the high levels of radiation emitted.

But a report by the UN's Committee on the Effects of Atomic Radiation (UNSCEAR) "concludes that there is no evidence of a major public health impact attributable to radiation exposure 14 years after the accident," the Vienna-based IAEA said.[234]

The myth persists anyway. The Associated Press recently reported, "The Ukrainian government blames the accident for at least 4,000 deaths among cleanup personnel and an elevated risk of disease among an estimated 3.4 million Ukrainians."[235]

The 1,800 child cancers are a tragedy. But the incidence of cancer has been tremendously exaggerated since the accident occurred. Chernobyl was a disaster of sorts, but not a catastrophe of mythical proportions.

Myth: Childhood Cancer Rates Are Rising

Exploiting our concerns for children, anti-chemical activists try to blame chemicals for a supposed epidemic of cancer in kids. Don't fall for it.

Cancer Rates for Children Worry Experts;
Hundreds Gather to Discuss Threat

declared the *San Francisco Chronicle* on September 17, 1997. The article continued:

A nation that has long celebrated the vanquishing of infectious diseases like smallpox, polio and measles as major killers of children now faces another ominous threat: a steady increase in childhood cancer.

Federal health and environmental experts gathered in Arlington, Va., this week to examine what environmental factors—from pesticides in food to pollutants in air and water—might be contributing to the steady increase in the disease over the past two decades.

The Environmental Protection Agency followed this conference with the publication of its *1998 Children's Environmental Health Yearbook*, which claimed, "The overall incidence rate of new cancers in children has increased [by about 12 percent from 1973 to 1994 in the United States]."[236] The yearbook's implication was that the increase was due to chemicals in the environment.

There are two issues here: (1) Is there an increase in cancer in children? (2) If there is an increase, are chemicals in the environment responsible?

First, some perspective is in order. Childhood cancer is pretty rare:

The overall annual incidence of cancer in U.S. children 0 to 14 years of age at diagnosis is 143.9 per million for white males and 126.9 per million for white females. The comparable incidence rate for black males and females is 107.2 and 107.9 per million, respectively. This is in contrast to 330.4 and 277.0 per 100,000 in white males and females, respectively, of all ages. The comparable figures for black males and females of all ages are 351.3 and 227.1 per 100,000, respectively. Thus, adult incidence of cancer (all ages) in the United States is over 20 times greater than the cancer incidence in children 0 to 14 years of age at diagnosis. The rarity issue becomes even more salient when one looks at the incidence of childhood cancers beyond acute leukemias and brain cancers. The U.S. annual incidence of all leukemia is 47.8 per million in white males and 29.5 per million in white females, and for brain and spinal tumors it is 26.4 and 23.3 in white male and female children, respectively. Thus, leukemias account for 51.6 and 49.5% of all cancers in 0- to 14-year-old white males and females, respectively. Once we go beyond these two cancer groups, other groups are more truly rare diseases. For example, the incidence of rhabdomyosarcoma (RMS) in children is 5.0 and 4.4 per million in white males and females, and that of osteosarcoma is 2.3 and 2.7 per million in white males and females, respectively. (References omitted)[237]

Childhood cancer does not appear to be on the rise.

- A study in the *Journal of the National Cancer Institute* reported: "As a childhood disease, cancer is rare, with 8,400 new cases expected in U.S. children ages 0 to 14 in 1999. However, it is the leading cause of death by disease in this age group, with 1,600 deaths expected this year. Since 1973, the incidence rate for cancer in children has changed little, but the death rate has declined about 50% from 1973 to 1995."[238]
- Because of public concern about possible increases in childhood cancer incidence in the United States, researchers examined recent incidence and mortality patterns for cancer in children. Their study, "Cancer Surveillance Series: Recent Trends in Childhood Cancer Incidence and Mortality in the United States," published in the *Journal of the National Cancer Institute*, reported: "There was no substantial change in incidence for the major pediatric cancers, and rates have remained relatively stable since the mid-1980s. The modest increases that were observed for brain/CNS cancers, leukemia, and infant neuroblastoma were confined to the mid-1980s. The patterns suggest that the increases likely reflected diagnostic improvements or reporting changes."[239]
- A recent study in the *Journal of the National Cancer Institute* examined the reported increase of 35 percent in primary malignant brain tumors among children in the United States during the period from 1973 through 1994.[240] The researchers concluded that the reported increase "resulted from changes in detection and/or reporting of childhood primary malignant brain tumors during the mid-1980s."
- "Since the early 1960s, the incidence of childhood cancers, and in particular childhood leukemia has remained relatively stable, or if anything has risen in geographic areas where there are adequate cancer registration systems," wrote researchers in the journal *Cancer*.[241]

Since the 1997 conference, the EPA appears to have backed off from the claim that childhood cancer is increasing, stating on its Web site, "The overall incidence rate of new cancers in children remains relatively unchanged." But the agency hasn't yielded on its claim that the environment is causing many of the cancers that do occur.

The EPA lists six possible causes of this cancer, including environmental tobacco smoke, radon, asbestos, ultraviolet light, hazardous waste, and some pesticides.[242] Unfortunately, there is no factual support for these allegations:

- *Environmental Tobacco Smoke*: The alleged link between exposure to secondhand smoke and cancer in adults is controversial—a federal judge even vacated the EPA's report linking secondhand smoke to cancers in adulthood because EPA manipulated the data to achieve its predetermined conclusion. The alleged link between ETS and childhood cancer is even more tenuous. A review of studies containing data on ETS and childhood cancer reported no statistical associations for "specific neoplasms such as leukemia (RR 1.05; CI, 0.82-1.34; 8 studies) and central nervous system tumors (RR 1.04; CI, 0.92-1.18, 12 studies). Results for other specific neoplasms were sparse, but the available data did not suggest a strong association for any type of tumor. No clear evidence of dose response was present in the studies that addressed this issue."

- *Radon:* Although adults with high occupational exposures to radon—e.g., underground uranium miners—have higher rates of lung cancer, children don't have such high-level exposures. Studies have reported no association between radon and children's acute myeloid leukemia[243] or central nervous system cancers.[244]

- *Asbestos:* The primary disease of overexposure to asbestos is mesothelioma. But "mesothelioma occurs rarely in children and . . . this diagnosis is difficult to establish. . . . Mesothelioma in children . . . is likely to have a multifactorial etiology. Radiation, prenatal medications, and genetic factors are all possible etiologic agents in childhood mesothelioma."[245]

- *Ultraviolet light:* Skin cancers, such as melanoma and basal cell carcinoma, occur rarely in children.[246] It's not clear whether these cancers are related to overexposure to sunlight.[247]
- *Hazardous Waste:* Studies have not linked childhood cancer with hazardous waste sites. A recent study of hazardous waste sites in North Carolina reported: "No significantly elevated cancer incidence rates were found at the county level. Two ZIP-code areas had statistically significant elevations in cancer incidence (p < .05). Only 3 of the cancer cases we mapped resided within a 1.6-km (1 mi) buffer zone of a National Priorities List hazardous-waste site. These 3 cases were not in the ZIP-code areas that had increased incidence rates."[248] Another recent study found no association between childhood cancer and 460 hazardous waste sites in the United Kingdom.[249]
- *Pesticides:* A critical review of 31 epidemiologic studies published between 1970 and 1996, which investigated whether occupational or residential exposure to pesticides of either parents or children was related to increased risk of childhood cancer, was unable to link pesticides with childhood cancer.[250]

So evidence indicates childhood cancer rates are stable, and no evidence indicates that chemicals or other substances in the environment are causing identifiable childhood cancers.

Myth: Children Are More Sensitive to Chemicals

Junk science exploitation of children includes the argument that children are more susceptible to danger from chemicals than are adults. The argument has intuitive appeal. "Children are not little adults," is the oft-heard sound bite.[251] Children certainly aren't little adults. But that does not mean that children are more susceptible than adults to harm from chemicals.[252] In fact, there is an extensive database on the pharmacokinetics of therapeutic drugs in infants and children. The elimination/clearance of many drugs is higher in children than in adults and this difference would apply to other xenobiotics. In consequence, children frequently will have lower body burdens than adults for the same daily intake of a chemical when this is expressed on a body weight basis, as used to describe the ADI (Acceptable Daily Intake) or TDI (Tolerable Daily Intake) (e.g. mg/kg body weight/day). Therefore, an increased safety or uncertainty factor for post-suckling infants and children is not required in relation to age-related differences in toxicokinetics. Indeed, the higher clearance of many xenobiotics (toxicokinetics) by children compared with adults may compensate, at least in part, for increased organ sensitivity (toxico-dynamics) during development.[253]

Children can be given near adult doses of the heart drug digoxin with less toxicity because they have a higher clearance of the drug.[254] Children at four months reportedly processed caffeine at the same rate as adults and then at higher rates later.[255] This is not to say that there aren't any exposures to which children are "more sensitive" than adults, but it's not true that children are more sensitive generally. Those that make this claim should be compelled to back it up with some sort of data.

Myth: DDT Causes Cancer

There's "original sin" and then there's "original junk science." That is the DDT scare. Rachel Carson sounded the alarm about the insecticide DDT in her book *Silent Spring*.[256] She alleged that DDT decimated bird populations and caused cancer in humans. Public fear over DDT was "validated" in 1972 when the Environmental Protection Agency banned virtually all uses of DDT. But Carson's concerns about DDT have yet to be justified, and the EPA's ban of DDT was based on politics, not science.

Carson predicted a cancer epidemic that could hit "practically 100 percent" of the human population. This prediction hasn't materialized, no doubt because it was based on a 1961 epidemic of liver cancer in middle-aged rainbow trout—later attributed to aflatoxin, a fungal toxin. There is no credible evidence whatsoever that DDT poses a cancer risk.[257]

The EPA administrative law judge who presided for seven months and 9,000 pages worth of testimony during the 1971–72 DDT ban hearings concluded:

> DDT is not a carcinogenic hazard to man. . . . DDT is not a mutagenic or teratogenic hazard to man. . . . The use of DDT under the regulations involved here does not have a deleterious effect on freshwater fish, estuarine organisms, wild birds or other wildlife.[258]

Despite the exculpatory ruling, then–EPA administrator William Ruckelshaus banned DDT anyway—and for less than scientific reasons.[259] Ruckelshaus never attended the hearings, did not read the transcript, and refused to release the materials used to make his decision. He even rebuffed a U.S. Department of Agriculture effort to obtain those materials through the Freedom of Information Act, claiming they were just "internal memos." It gets worse.

Ruckelshaus made no secret of his bias against DDT. As a member of the activist group the Environmental Defense Fund, Ruckelshaus later solicited donations for EDF on personal stationery that read, "EDF's scientists blew the whistle on DDT by showing it to be a cancer hazard, and three years later, when the dust had cleared, EDF had won." Yes, it did. Thanks to the Ruckelshaus Railroad.

Myth: Low-Level Lead Exposure Lowers IQ

Greater Dangers for Young Children
Indicated in Study on Lead Effects

headlined the *Washington Post* on March 29, 1979. The article continued:

> Amounts of lead well below those previously considered hazardous can adversely affect the intelligence and school behavior of young children, according to a study published in today's edition of the *New England*

Journal of Medicine. The study, which involved 3,329 children in the Boston area, has serious implications for children in the District of Columbia and other urban areas, local officials said yesterday.

In 1977, 15 percent of the children screened in Washington for lead poisoning had lead levels in their bodies equal to or above those of the children in the study's "high lead" group. The study, by Dr. Herbert Needleman of Harvard University Medical School and Boston Children's Hospital, compared the IQs of 58 "high lead" levels. The study also includes analyses by teachers of the learning abilities and behavior of the children.

All children in the study were first and second-grade students in Chelsea and Somerville, Mass., outside Boston. According to the study, the "high-lead" group had a mean IQ of 102.1, compared to the "low lead" group's mean of 106.6. The teachers perceived even more dramatic differences in the behaviors of the two groups, with 26 percent of the "high lead" group rated as unable to follow a sequence of directions, while only 8 percent of the "low-lead" children were in that category.

The news propelled concerns about low-level exposures to lead and researcher Herbert Needleman into national prominence:

> Needleman has testified for Congress; consulted for the Environmental Protection Agency (EPA), the Centers for Disease Control, and the Agency for Toxic Substances and Disease registry; and is a major author of government policy documents. He has testified for plaintiffs in many tort cases in which children have claimed damages as a result of lead exposure. He has obtained grant support from [the National Institutes of Health] and EPA to conduct further research on this topic. In *Science*, he was called the "Get-the-Lead-Out Guru." . . . Needleman's activities have been important in setting federal policies that will be very costly.[260]

But researchers discovered a variety of problems with Needleman's research.[261] He didn't control for the confounding factor of a child's age—factoring in age yielded few significant results. Needleman excluded children who were "lead poisoned" but did not have impaired intelligence. Other results that did not support Needleman's conclusions were not reported.

A panel convened by the EPA to assist in preparing a revision of the air quality standard for lead concluded,

In summary, at this time, based on questionable [lead] exposure categorization and subject exclusion methods, problems with missing data, and concerns regarding the statistical analyses employed and selected for reporting, the Committee concludes that the study results, as reported in the Needleman paper, neither support nor refute the hypothesis that low or moderate levels of [lead] exposure lead to cognitive or other behavioral impairments in children.[262]

Needleman was subsequently accused of scientific misconduct because of the study. The University of Pittsburgh inquiry panel that reviewed Needleman's study reported,

Based on the subject selection and classification problems alone it is doubtful whether [Needleman's study] represents a fair and accurate ascertainment of the relationship between IQ and dentine levels [among the study subjects]. The panel recommends that a full investigation be held to determine if the apparent inappropriate selection of cases and incomplete presentations of results constitutes research misconduct.[263]

Needleman was ultimately found not guilty of scientific misconduct. But as this letter in the *New England Journal of Medicine* points out, Needleman and his study were hardly vindicated.

The investigative bodies (the University of Pittsburgh and the federal Office of Research Integrity) found Needleman's studies scientifically flawed. Both investigative groups described Needleman's work as involving a "pattern of errors, omissions, contradictions and incomplete information from the original publications to the present." The University of Pittsburgh found that Needleman had engaged in "deliberate misrepresentation" and "substandard science"; they referred to Needleman's dismissal of critics as lead industry representatives and to his attempts to intimidate his investigators, including the university board itself. The university's report stated that had Needleman accurately described his methodology and subject selection, he "would have risked rejection" of his article by the *New England Journal of Medicine*. In addition, the Office of Research Integrity cited misplotted graph points, which were found "difficult to explain as honest error," and uncorrected mistakes in Needleman's original *New England Journal of Medicine* manuscript pointed out by a coauthor.[264]

So is low-level lead exposure in children associated with reduced IQ?

A systematic review of 26 epidemiological studies since 1979 concluded that a "doubling of body lead burden (from 10 to 20 micrograms/deciliter blood lead or from 5 to 10 micrograms per gram of tooth lead) is [statistically] associated with a mean deficit in full-scale IQ of around 1-2 IQ points."[265] But the authors add,

> While low level lead exposure may cause a small IQ deficit, other explanations need considering: are the published studies representative; is there inadequate allowance for confounders; are there selection biases in recruiting and following children; and do children of lower IQ adopt behaviour which makes them more prone to lead uptake (reverse causality)?

Translation? If there is an association between lead and IQ, it's too small to measure.

Myth: Love Canal Was an Environmental Disaster

When the Love Canal controversy began in August 1978, the Associated Press reported:

> New York State will evacuate 35 families from an area contaminated by decades-old chemicals, the state health commissioner said. . . . The state Health Department had recommended that pregnant women and families with children younger than 2 years old be evacuated from the area. The department said it found the rate of miscarriages in the area was 50 percent higher than the national average. It also noted several instances of birth defects.
>
> Air monitors placed in local residences by the federal Environmental Protection Agency have recorded concentrations of some chemicals 250 to 5,000 times levels considered to be safe. . . . Hooker Chemical Corp. had dumped chemicals in the area between 1930 and 1953, when it was covered over and sold to the city, which later sold plots of land for residential development. State researchers have found that 82 separate chemicals, stored underground in drums, have begun seeping to the surface.
>
> According to area residents, the chemicals first began surfacing in 1976 after several seasons of abnormally heavy rains. Some residents said chemicals have seeped through the walls of their basements.[266]

And while there is no question that chemical waste seeping through basement walls is undesirable, the health consequences turned out to be a lot less than the hype.

The alleged 50 percent increase in miscarriage was not a scientific study. It was only a collection of anecdotes collected from interviews with residents.[267] Hype outpaced science at Love Canal entirely.

"A bibliography about Love Canal cited more than 500 documents. Of these, only three that dealt with health effects were to citations in peer-reviewed journals, " wrote Philip Abelson, editor of *Science*, in 1985.[268] Here are the results of the three studies:

- A weak statistical association was reported for low–birth weight babies and residence in the historic swale area from 1940 through 1953, the period when various chemicals were dumped in this disposal site.[269] But there was no association reported for the period 1954 through 1978 when people actually lived over the waste site, the trigger for the panic. The authors also acknowledged: "It is important to emphasize that the low birth weight data used for all analyses were obtained from birth records and not through interview. There are several major difficulties in study design that limit the interpretation of results. It is not certain that all infants born in the area during the study period were included in this investigation. Although it is clear that human exposure to a specific toxic agent can result in an adverse reproductive outcome, it is exceedingly difficult to define exposure in multichemical settings such as the Love Canal. In addition, the evidence associating low birth weight with toxic chemical exposure is limited. Other variables, for which there are no objective data, can influence the frequency of the end point. Although we found no convincing evidence that educational level, smoking, occupation, past medical or therapeutic histories influenced the results, most of these data were obtained from interviews and are, therefore, subject to recall bias. In addition, it was impossible to examine other important variables such as alcohol ingestion before and during the pregnancies included in this study."[270]

- No differences in chromosomal aberrations were reported between Love Canal residents, including those in whose homes levels of chemicals spreading from the waste dump were measured, and controls.[271]

- "Data from the New York Cancer Registry show no evidence for higher cancer rates associated with residence near the Love Canal toxic waste burial site in comparison with the entire state outside of New York City. Rates of liver cancer, lymphoma, and leukemia, which were selected for special attention, were not consistently elevated. Among the other cancers studied, a higher rate was noted only for respiratory cancer, but it was not consistent across age groups and appeared to be related to a high rate for the entire city of Niagara Falls. There was no evidence that the lung cancer rate was associated with the toxic wastes buried at the dump site."[272]

Love Canal remains a rallying point for environmental activists—as if repeating the myth makes it so.

Myth: Three Mile Island Was a Nuclear Disaster

Who could forget the "nuclear disaster" that occurred at the Three Mile Island nuclear power plant? Certainly not readers of the *Dallas Morning News* or viewers of *ABC World News Tonight*, examples of media that still refer to the events at Three Mile Island as a "nuclear disaster."[273] But was it a "disaster"?

On March 28, 1979, a pressure relief valve became stuck open at the Three Mile Island Unit-2 reactor, releasing radiation into the surrounding area. According to a report by the U.S. Nuclear Regulatory Commission (NRC), the average dose of radiation received by the

2 million people in the surrounding area was 0.0014 rem. A rem is a measurement unit for absorbed radiation dose in man. The average member of the U.S. population receives about 0.36 rem of radiation annually from naturally occurring radiation, medical uses of radiation, and consumer products. The highest estimated individual exposure resulting from the Three Mile Island release was 0.075 rem.

A number of people claimed in a lawsuit that they developed cancer as a result of exposure to the radiation released during the incident. The plaintiffs contended that they were exposed to 100 rems of radiation, not the measly 0.0014 rem estimated by the NRC. In ruling against the plaintiffs, the court acknowledged that the plaintiffs were clearly exposed to radiation released by the Three Mile Island incident, but they failed to present evidence that they were exposed to enough radiation to cause their cancers.

Although the plaintiffs claimed over 100 rems of exposure—a level experienced by some of the survivors of the atomic bomb explosion at Hiroshima—the court noted that, to win, they would only have to present evidence of exposure to 10 rems of radiation. Still, the plaintiffs failed to produce evidence of even this exposure level. The court stated:

> The parties have had nearly two decades to muster evidence in support of their respective cases. . . . The paucity of proof alleged in support of the Plaintiffs' case is manifest. The court searched for any and all evidence which construed in a light most favorable to Plaintiffs' case creates a genuine issue of material fact warranting submission of the claims to a jury. This effort has been in vain.

The most recent study reports no increase in cancer or death rates among the 32,135 residents near Three Mile Island.[274]

As it turns out, the Three Mile Island incident was not a disaster for the surrounding population. But it was for the rest of us. Three Mile Island doomed the nuclear power industry and ended (for the foreseeable future) the prospect of cheap and clean electric power in this country.

Myth Universe

This wasn't a comprehensive presentation of the myth universe, which, like the real universe, is immense and ever expanding. Don't expect to learn the entire myth universe. That would easily take a Ph.D.-level effort.

Since myths are simply rehashed health scares, deal with myths the same way you learned in Lesson 2 to deal with new health scares—"Show Me the Science!"

LESSON 11:
TRICKS ARE FOR KIDS

It is true that you may fool all of the people some
of the time;
you can even fool some of the people all of the time;
but you can't fool all of the people all of the time.

—Abraham Lincoln

THE FUNDAMENTAL SKILLS of Junk Science Judo will serve you well in debunking any health scare. But you will need to know some oft-used tricks of the junk science trade.

Rule: You Can't Prove a Negative
In science, the burden of proof is on the researcher trying to advance a theory. But junk scientists turn this burden upside down. Instead of demonstrating through the scientific method that a substance or condition is dangerous, the junk science mob demands that the substance or condition be proven absolutely safe.

This reversal of the burden of proof is called the "precautionary principle." The ostensible motivation behind the principle is "better safe than sorry." While the precautionary principle has some initial intuitive appeal, it has a potentially fatal defect. If the precautionary principle is imposed in an absolute manner—requiring proof that something will never be dangerous to anyone under any circumstances—then it becomes the logical fallacy of "proving a negative"—proving the nonexistence of that for which no evidence of any kind exists.[275]

Illogical Fallout

"A program that pays up to $100,000 to people sickened by Cold War–era uranium mining and nuclear tests will be dramatically expanded under a bill signed by President Clinton," reported the Associated Press in July 2000. The article explained:

> The changes augment a 1990 law giving payments to . . . "downwinders"—people who lived in areas most affected by nuclear fallout from tests—with cancers or other ailments linked to their radiation exposure. . . . The aim is to compensate those unknowingly exposed to radiation while working to develop the U.S. nuclear arsenal from World War II until 1971. . . . Above-ground nuclear tests in New Mexico and Nevada spread radioactive fallout across broad areas of the Southwest.
>
> "The president believes that people who have gotten sick from radioactive fallout . . . should not have to jump through unnecessary hoops to be compensated," [the White House said].

The article omitted mention of the lack of evidence that the so-called downwinders had been affected by fallout. A 10-year, $18 million study conducted by the Centers for Disease Control and Prevention failed to identify an association between exposure to fallout and thyroid disease, the health effect of concern with radioactive fallout.[276]

But in December 1999 the chairman of a panel of the National Research Council said: "We agree with the investigators that the study provides no clear evidence of an association between levels of people's exposure to radioactive iodine and their rates of thyroid diseases. However, given both the statistical uncertainties in the data and the uncertainties associated with the estimated radiation doses to the thyroid, we do not believe a strong statement can be made that there is no association."[277]

So the NRC chairman wanted the CDC to prove the negative—that no association existed between exposure to fallout and thyroid disease. This is quite impossible, especially since an association could exist just by chance.

If the precautionary principle is used in a "reasonable" manner, on the other hand, then scientists are quite capable of designing tests to determine whether a substance or condition is reasonably safe. Such tests are the basis for the setting of safety standards for exposure to substances and conditions by government regulatory agencies.

A Cautionary Tale

The European Union wants to apply the precautionary principle in the absolute sense. Members of the EU have used the precautionary principle to close their markets to imports that compete with local industries. The EU has shut out Canadian and U.S. beef, claiming that meat from hormone-treated cattle may cause cancer. The EU wants to exclude genetically modified foods from the United States and Canada, asserting that health and environmental consequences are unknown and potentially significant. There is also internecine use of the principle among EU members. France and Germany are fighting to keep out British beef because of their concerns about "mad cow" disease.

In none of these cases does scientific evidence lend credence to the ostensible concerns. Yet science cannot prove the absolute safety of meat from hormone-treated cattle, biotechnology foods, or beef. Bear in mind that science cannot prove the safety of "organic" or "natural" foods either.

The EU's use of the precautionary principle is quite cynical. David Byrne, the EU's health and consumer protection commissioner, said at the 1999 World Trade Organization meeting in Seattle, "Our [trade] partners should know that our decisions are not arbitrary and disguised protectionism."[278] But in the preceding week Byrne had imposed an emergency ban on soft plastic toys containing a class of chemicals called phthalates. The ban ignored the unanimous advice of the EU's scientific committee, which said there was no evidence of danger to children.

"Better safe than sorry" is not science.

Rule: Meta-analysis Is a House of Cards

Ever try to stand a playing card up on its edge? It's pretty tough. But you can take a deck of cards and build a house of cards. That's the kind of house you build when you use the statistical technique called meta-analysis. Meta-analysis takes individual studies that don't stand up on their own from a statistical point of view and combines their statistics to construct a new statistically stronger and newsworthy study.

We often find numerous epidemiologic studies on a given topic with varying and conflicting results—typically involving weak associations. Good examples are the approximately 40 studies on secondhand smoke and lung cancer. Some studies report a positive weak statistical association between secondhand smoke and lung cancer. Others report no statistical association. Some even report a negative correlation.

The existence of such a variety of weak association results indicates one of two things: either there is no association between secondhand smoke and lung cancer or the association is so small that it cannot be reliably detected and quantified.

Unhappy with those outcomes, though, the Junksters resorted to meta-analysis.

Secondhand Smoke Peril Affirmed; EPA Move to Endorse Report on Cigarettes May Affect Workplace

headlined the *Washington Post* in January 1993. The article continued,

> In a long-delayed decision that eventually could have a major impact on the American workplace, the Environmental Protection Agency will conclude officially Thursday that exposure to "secondhand" cigarette

smoke causes lung cancer in adults and greatly increases the risk of respiratory illnesses in children.[279]

The *Washington Post* and the *Los Angeles Times* were the only media outlets to note the EPA's use of meta-analysis in arriving at the conclusion about secondhand smoke. Neither offered a critical explanation of the technique.[280] But times have changed—a little, anyway. A meta-analysis published in the *New England Journal of Medicine* in 1999 attempted to link secondhand smoke with increased risk of heart disease.[281] But there were fewer headlines than there had been for the EPA report in 1993. The few headlines that appeared explain why.

On March 25, 1999, for example, the (*New Orleans*) *Times Picayune* reported

Secondhand Smoke Tied to Heart Ills;
but Researchers' Technique Slammed

The article continued:

> In a computer-driven study of more than 640,000 people, Tulane University researchers found that long-term exposure to tobacco smoke can raise a nonsmoker's risk of developing coronary heart disease by 25 percent. . . .
>
> But the article is drawing fire—in the same publication. In an editorial, University of Chicago Hospitals health studies Chairman John Bailar [a highly distinguished statistician] attacks everything about the study, from the researchers' methods to the data upon which they relied. . . . The report stirred anew the debate about meta-analysis, an evolving tool that was impossible before computers let scientists analyze studies involving vast numbers of people.
>
> For their inquiry, Whelton and his colleagues conducted a computer-based survey of 18 earlier investigations of the effects of passive smoking involving 643,750 people.
>
> In his editorial, Bailar assailed this approach, saying it is "no reliable substitute for epidemiologic research." "I regretfully conclude that we still do not know, with accuracy, how much or even whether exposure to environmental tobacco smoke increases the risk of coronary heart disease," he wrote.

Bailar's editorial warrants special attention.

> Can meta-analysis of epidemiologic studies on this topic provide a more reliable conclusion than a thoughtful review of the usual type? There are reasons to think that it cannot.
>
> The first reason is the quality of the data. Most studies of lung cancer and [secondhand smoke] likewise reported a positive association, and those findings have been received with some skepticism because of concern about the quality of the data. Among the reasons for concern are a possible tendency of nonsmokers with lung cancer to look for some external reason (for instance, smoking by a spouse or coworker) for an otherwise inexplicable disease, inaccuracies in the reporting of exposure to environmental tobacco smoke, and reluctance to report a personal history of smoking. [These researchers] gave little consideration to such possible problems with the quality of the studies they analyzed. Surely not all those studies were perfect.
>
> A second reason for concern is the procedure for meta-analysis itself. The published literature on some topics may reflect the greater likelihood of publication of positive results than of negative results. . . .
>
> The authors do not comment on the remarkable uniformity of the findings of the 18 studies, despite the large variations in study design, methods, and populations. For example, if environmental tobacco smoke causes coronary heart disease, why are estimates of this effect from studies that include exposure in the workplace about the same as those from studies that do not?. . . A great deal of uniformity among the results of independent studies of a particular phenomenon is not necessarily good: it can suggest consistency in bias rather than consistency in real effects.[282]

What a difference an explanation makes.

Rule: Pooling Is Fooling

Meta-analysis is a trick collapsing many statistically weak studies into one statistically stronger study. An analogy within a single epidemiologic study is to collapse different statistical categories into one category to achieve a stronger statistical result. It's a little like averaging numbers or grades. All it takes is one unusually "high" number to drag up the statistically insignificant numbers.

Uniting States for Gun Control

Gun Laws Credited with Drop in Deaths; Fewer Children Killed by Accidental Gunfire, Local Researchers Find

headlined the *Seattle Times* in October 1997. The article continued:

> In states with felony laws requiring safe gun storage, accidental deaths of children by gunfire have dropped more than 40 percent, Seattle researchers have found. A study by physicians at the Harborview Injury Prevention and Research Center showed, however, that there was no change in the deaths where laws allow only misdemeanor prosecutions for such violations.
>
> Reported in tomorrow's edition of the *Journal of the American Medical Association*, the study comes as campaigning intensifies for Initiative 676 in Washington state. Among its provisions, the measure would require trigger locks on all handguns sold or transferred.
>
> The study, which looked at all 12 states that have safe-storage laws, is the first since Florida passed the initial measure in 1989. When the states were lumped together, there were 23 percent fewer unintentional deaths than would be expected, considering nationwide trends.
>
> "This is the best evidence of the effectiveness of these laws. It looks like they work," said Dr. Peter Cummings, study director and an epidemiologist at the injury center and the University of Washington.

The study is frequently cited by gun control advocates, such as Handgun Control, Inc. "A 1997 study published in the *Journal of American Medical Association* found that state safe storage laws are particularly effective at reducing gun injuries and deaths among children," according to Handgun Control, Inc.[283] But a closer analysis of the study reveals that the reduction in deaths was attributable largely to the experience in one state and that there was no consistent beneficial effect in the other states.[284] If safe storage laws were truly effective, the reduction in deaths likely would show up in more states, no?

All for Junk, and Junk for All

Study Finds High Exposure to Dioxin Increases Cancer Risk

reported the Associated Press on May 5, 1999. The article continued:

> Chemical workers exposed to high levels of dioxin have a 60 percent increased chance of dying of cancer, but the chemical poses no added cancer risk to the general population, a study says. Kyle Steenland, co-author of the study appearing today in the *Journal of the National Cancer Institute*, said the research suggests most people typically are not exposed to dangerous levels of dioxin and that cancer appears to result only among those who had extremely high and long-term exposures to the chemical 15 to 20 years ago.
>
> "There is not a significant increase in cancers until you get to the upper" exposure levels, Steenland said Tuesday. "This is not raising a red flag by saying that low level exposure is causing a lot of cancer."

The researcher's conclusion is based on a pooling of the *weak* statistical associations for specific cancers into a category called "all cancers." Check out the study's results for "all cancers" and specific cancer sites in Table 11.1.[285]

You'll notice that other than the statistical associations for bladder and larynx cancers, none of the reported statistical associations is statistically significant by virtue of its confidence intervals. (We don't know about the *p*-values because they weren't reported—or do we?)

The researchers try to circumvent this problem by combining data for the specific cancer sites into an "all cancer" category. But as Bruce Charlton pointed out earlier:

> The root of most instances of statistical malpractice is the breaking of mathematical neutrality and the introduction of causal assumptions into the analysis without scientific grounds. This amounts to performing science by sleight-of-hand: the quickness of statistics deceives the mind.

In this case, the researchers assumed that it was biologically possible for dioxin to be a cancer-causing agent at all sites in the body—even though there is really no persuasive evidence that it acts as a cancer-

Table 11.1: Dioxin and Cancer

Type of Cancer	No. of Deaths	SMR (95% CI)
All cancers	377	1.13 (1.02–1.25)
Esophagus	13	1.46 (0.77–2.49)
Stomach	13	1.04 (0.55–1.78)
Small intestine, colon	34	1.16 (0.80–1.61)
Rectum	6	0.85 (0.31–1.85)
Liver and biliary	7	0.88 (0.44–1.57)
Pancreas	16	0.96 (0.55–1.56)
Peritoneum and unspecified	3	2.19 (0.45–6.41)
Larynx	10	2.22 (1.06–4.08)
Lung	125	1.06 (0.88–1.26)
Prostate	28	1.17 (0.78–1.69)
Kidney	13	1.56 (0.82–2.66)
Bladder	16	1.99 (1.13–3.23)
Lymphatic and hematopoietic	35	1.11 (0.78–1.54)
Hodgkin's disease	3	1.09 (0.22–3.19)
Non-Hodgkin's lymphoma	12	1.10 (0.56–1.91)
Multiple myeloma	10	2.07 (0.99–3.80)
Leukemia and aleukemia	10	0.81 (0.38–1.48)
Brain and nervous system	8	0.81 (0.35–1.60)
Connective tissue and soft tissue	4	2.32 (0.63–5.93)

causing agent at even one site. The "all cancers" category is a statistical trick to enable the conclusion that dioxin is a cancer-causing substance.

A general rule that may be taken from the "all cancers" trick is, in epidemiologic studies, beware of statistical pooling intended to overcome data that provide the "wrong" answer.

Rule: Buck the Trend Analysis
Some researchers try to overcome weak and nonsignificant relative risks by showing "trends" of the relative risks. These trends usually involve the so-called dose-response relationship—the change in rate

of disease as compared to the change in exposure rate. Under traditional toxicology theory, disease rates generally increase with increasing exposure to the substance or condition of interest.

But don't be fooled. Like meta-analysis, trend analysis is just another statistical trick to try to make something out of nothing.

On August 19, 1998, the *Los Angeles Times* reported

High Selenium Levels May Ward Off Cancer

The article continued:

> Eating foods rich in the trace mineral selenium may help men ward off advanced prostate cancer, a new report suggests. A study of 33,737 men found that "higher selenium levels were associated with a reduced risk of advanced prostate cancer," researchers from Harvard University in Cambridge, Mass., report in the Journal of the National Cancer Institute. Prostate cancer causes nearly 40,000 deaths annually in the U.S. Selenium is found in minute amounts in meat, fish, whole grains, dairy products and vegetables grown in selenium-rich soil.[286]

The researchers reported a statistically significant trend for a decrease in the occurrence of advanced prostate cancer with increasing consumption of selenium.[287] They classified selenium consumption into quintiles (Quintile 1 = lowest 20 percent in consumption of selenium, Quintile 5 = highest 20 percent in consumption). The study's relative risks and 95 percent confidence intervals are presented in Table 11.2. Note that the relative risks for Quintile 2 and Quintile 4 are not statistically significant because the upper bounds of their confidence

Table 11.2: Relative Risk and 95 Percent Confidence Intervals

	Quintile of Selenium Consumption					
	1	2	3	4	5	*p* for Trend
RR	1.0	0.59	0.35	0.76	0.35	0.03
(95% CI)	(Reference)	(0.27–1.30)	(0.16–0.78)	(0.34–1.73)	(0.16–0.78)	

intervals are greater than 1.0. So only Quintile 3 and Quintile 5 report reduced rates of prostate cancer. Some trend, huh? Two noncontiguous data points that are the same. But for the researchers—who ignore the lack of statistically significant data points—it's a trend!

Study Shows Dangers of Stick Margarine and Shortening

reported the Associated Press on November 19, 1997. The article continued:

> Ordinary stick margarine, as well as anything baked and fried with shortening and other kinds of hardened vegetable oil, appear to be the worst foods of all for the heart. A large new study offers the strongest evidence yet that something called trans fat, which is a primary ingredient of standard stick margarine and shortening, is an especially unhealthy part of the diet.

The researchers reported a statistically significant trend (Table 11.3) for an increase in heart disease rates with increasing consumption of so-called trans fats.[288]

This is even worse than the selenium example. Three of the four data points in the "trend" are not statistically significant. What kind of trend has two data points? This type of trend analysis can only be explained as an effort to sidestep data that don't fit the junk science agenda.

Table 11.3: Heart Disease and Trans Fats

	Quintile of Trans Fat Consumption					
	1	2	3	4	5	p for Trend
RR	1.0	1.09	1.16	1.24	1.53	0.002
(95%CI)	(Reference)	(0.87–1.37)	(0.91–1.47)	(0.96–1.60)	(1.16–2.02)	

Rule: Results Should Match the Conclusion

Call me picky, but I like a study's conclusion to match the results.

Banned Pesticide, Breast Cancer Link Drawn

blared the *Boston Globe* on December 4, 1998. The article continued:

> A long-banned pesticide increases the risk of breast cancer, a study suggests, reviving a debate over the potential hazards of chemicals that mimic the hormone estrogen. In the study, published in this week's issue of the *Lancet*, a British medical journal, researchers found that women with the highest traces of the pesticide Dieldrin in their blood were twice as likely as women with the lowest levels to develop breast cancer.

Although the study reported a relative risk of only about 2.0 for blood levels of dieldrin and breast cancer, I was interested in the *Globe*'s comment that "blood samples were taken from the women in 1976 to check for levels of 48 pesticides. . . ." So what happened to the results for the other 47 pesticides? I obtained a copy of the study to see for myself.

The researchers undertook the study to see whether manmade organochlorine chemicals, including some pesticides and PCBs, were associated with increased rates of breast cancer. That was their hypothesis. They identified a population of more than 7,700 women who gave blood samples in 1976. Data on breast cancer incidence among the women were collected for the next 17 years. The researchers analyzed blood samples from the 240 women who eventually developed breast cancer.[289] Of the 48 tests, only the test for dieldrin produced a statistically significant association with breast cancer. The researchers concluded (incredibly),

> These findings support the hypothesis that exposure to [manmade organochlorine compounds] may increase the risk of breast cancer.

But how? Just by chance alone, one would expect about two statistically significant associations to be produced by so many tests.

The researchers didn't even do as well as chance. The absence of any other statistically significant associations among the other 47 organochlorine compounds and breast cancer doesn't say much for the biological plausibility of the dieldrin association.

A November 1992 study published in the *Journal of the National Cancer Institute* reported no statistical association between secondhand smoke and lung cancer among women living with a smoker who smoked one pack per day for 40 years or less.[290] Women who lived with a pack-a-day smoker for 40 or more years reportedly had a statistically nonsignificant 30 percent increase in lung cancer incidence.

Despite these "nonresults," the researchers concluded: "[Our study suggests] a small but consistent increased risk of lung cancer from passive smoking. Comprehensive actions to limit smoking in public places and worksites are well-advised." What?

The lead researcher did redeem himself somewhat in a subsequent newspaper interview in which he said:

> I wish our findings had gone in the exact pattern the public health community would like. But one of the criticisms of medical research is that the only thing findings ever show is some kind of health risk. I feel it's important to publish findings, no matter what they show.[291]

From his mouth to his own ears.

Rule: Regulatory Levels Are Safer Than Safe

Government regulatory agencies are responsible for setting standards for public and worker exposures to potentially hazardous substances and conditions. The standards are usually far more stringent than warranted by available scientific data.

In touting its January 1998 report "Overexposed: Organophosphate Insecticides in Children's Food," the Environmental Working Group stated,

> Every day, 1 million American children age 5 and under consume unsafe levels of a class of pesticides that can harm the developing brain and nervous system, according to a new analysis of federal data.[292]

But the EWG, an environmental activist group, did no analysis of safety. The study was based on levels of pesticide residues permitted in food by the Environmental Protection Agency. The levels—called "reference doses," or RfDs—may be set hundreds and even thousands of times lower than levels of pesticides reported to cause health effects in laboratory animals. RfD levels are set so low to provide wide margins of safety. If "safe" levels instead of RfDs had been used by the EWG, its conclusion probably would have been that no child is exposed to "unsafe" levels of pesticides.

Once, even the established regulatory level wasn't good enough for the EWG. So it made up its own. In touting its August 1997 report "Tough to Swallow: How Pesticide Companies Profit from Poisoning America's Tap Water," the EWG stated,

> For the past twenty-five years, maybe longer, millions of people living in hundreds of midwestern communities have been routinely drinking tap water contaminated with an unhealthy dose of agricultural weed killers, many of which are carcinogens.[293]

The federal permitted exposure level for the herbicide atrazine in drinking water was 3 parts per billion. But the EWG based its report on a standard of 0.15 parts per billion. In response to the report, an official from the Ohio EPA said, "We're concerned when reports like this come out because they're making comparisons based on levels that don't exist."[294]

Anti-pesticide activists target regulatory levels that make it possible for pesticides to be used. The only regulatory level acceptable to them is one that makes pesticide use impractical.

Rule: Don't Take a Long Walk off a Short "Peer Review"

The junk science mob often tries to bolster the credibility of a study by describing it as having been "peer reviewed"—the equivalent of scientific quality control. You're supposed to be comforted by the fact that other experts have reviewed the paper before publication and given it the green light. Peer review, however, does not guarantee that a study is good or valid. In fact, it is obvious that peer review isn't very effective at all—just consider all the junk science that is routinely published, even in the most prestigious journals. Peer review has two primary shortcomings:

- *Glorified Editing*: Reviewers typically see the study in its near final form and they typically don't receive or evaluate study data. They may spend (at most) a couple of hours reading and considering a study. Such reviews are not terribly thorough. The primary benefit of this type of review is that glaringly stupid mistakes are caught and corrected.

- *Rubber-Stamping*: Peer review is (unfortunately) not usually an adversarial process. Many journals are not looking to have articles shot down; they want to catch obvious problems and bolster study credibility. Oftentimes, the peer reviewers are colleagues of or otherwise sympathetic to the principal scientists.

    Evidence of the close connection of scientists was presented by scientists who adapted the game "Six Degrees of Kevin Bacon" to scientific researchers. The game posits that we are all connected by six or fewer stages of circumstance or acquaintance. Alfred Hitchcock can be linked to Bacon in three steps: Alfred Hitchcock was in *Show Business at War* (1943) with Orson Welles, and Orson Welles was in *A Safe Place* (1971) with Jack Nicholson, and Jack Nicholson was in *A Few Good Men* (1992) with Kevin Bacon.[295]

    The researchers determined that "scientific communities seem to constitute a 'small world,'" with only five or six steps needed to connect one randomly chosen scientist in a community to another.[296] Small communities of researchers may lead to similar (as opposed to independent) thinking and reluctance to criticize others in the community.

Former *New England Journal of Medicine* editor Arnold Relman said:

> Almost anything people want to publish, if it's not grossly in error or grossly untrue, will get published somewhere. Obviously, we are all interested in the truth, but it is mostly what happens after a study is published that determines the truth.[297]

He's right. It's the review of a study after publication that counts—not the cursory editing and rubber-stamping of a few friendly reviewers.

Implying that a study is valid because it has been peer reviewed is another effort to get you to overlook the quality of a study and its data. It's like getting you to buy a used car on the basis of the salesperson's recommendation, without checking under the hood and test driving it. You wouldn't do that, would you?

Rule: Beware of Risky Language

Journalists usually present the results of epidemiologic studies in terms of "risk." But you know now that epidemiology has little to do with risk (see Lesson 4: Epidemiology Is Statistics).

Breast Cancer: The Pill Raises Risk
in Women with Family History

headlined the Associated Press on October 10, 2000. The article continued:

> Birth control pills may raise the already heightened risk of breast cancer faced by women with a strong family history of the disease, a study suggests. Among sisters and daughters of women with breast cancer, users of the pill were three times more likely than nonusers to get the disease.
>
> And if at least five family members had breast or ovarian cancer, pill users faced an 11-fold risk, the researchers reported in Wednesday's Journal of the American Medical Association.

A correct report on the study would have read:

Use of birth control pills *was statistically associated with a higher rate* of breast cancer *among a small population of* women with a strong family history of the disease, a study *reports.*

Among sisters and daughters in 426 families of women diagnosed with breast cancer between 1944 and 1952 at the University of Minnesota Hospital, users of the pill *had three times more breast cancer* than nonusers.

Among sisters and daughters of women with breast cancer in the 35 families that had a history of five or more breast and ovarian cancers, pill users *had 11 times more breast cancer,* the researchers reported in Wednesday's *Journal of the American Medical Association.*

Though the Associated Press's "risk" language is more interesting and less cumbersome to read, it's simply wrong.

The researchers compared rates of breast cancer only among a small, select sample of birth control pill users. They did not causally link birth control pill use with breast cancer. The clinical causes of the reported breast cancers were not determined. This study shed no light on anyone's risk of breast cancer.

Giving journalists the benefit of the doubt—that they actually realize that epidemiology has nothing to do with risk—writing in terms of "risk" is either laziness or an attempt to make dull statistics more interesting.

Rule: Read the Study, Pass on the News

After you take in a news story on some new study or report, you might want to check out the actual study.

Cancer Risk from Air Pollution Still High, Study Says

reported the *Los Angeles Times* on March 1, 1999. The article continued:

Despite improved air quality in the Los Angeles Basin, residents still are breathing unusually dangerous levels of cancer-causing pollutants, according to a groundbreaking congressional study set to be released today.

Although California has made strides in reducing hazardous air pollution, the report found toxics at high enough levels that the risk of cancer was 426 times higher than health standards established by the 1990 federal Clean Air Act.

"We were surprised at the findings," said Rep. Henry A. Waxman (D-Los Angeles), who requested the report, prepared by the minority staff of the House Government Reform Committee. "They are so much higher than they ought to be."

Although data about air quality have long been available, experts say the study is the first of its kind to determine cancer risks in the air people actually breathe. Using thousands of air samples collected over the last three years at sites in Los Angeles, Long Beach and Burbank, the study computed and analyzed the health risks posed by various specific pollutants. . . .

Wallerstein said that since the Clean Air Act was adopted in 1990, cancer risks from toxic pollutants have been reduced by 40%. But the new AQMD data show lifetime risks of getting cancer from the air at levels 200 to 400 times higher than the Clean Air Act's health goals of one additional cancer case per million.

Frightening stuff—until you read the actual report, which states:

While the results of this study show a significant exposure to hazardous air pollutants in Los Angeles, there are several important caveats that should be considered in interpreting the estimates of health risks.

First, there is considerable scientific uncertainty about the cancer risk estimates for hazardous air pollutants. Most of the cancer risk estimates for these compounds are based on animal studies which have used high doses of the compounds. EPA uses conservative assumptions in extrapolating risks from animals to humans and from high to low doses. The risk estimates presented in this report therefore represent what could be described as the "upper bounds" of the risk. Moreover, the hazardous air pollutants examined in this analysis have, in general, not been as well studied as ozone, carbon monoxide, and other "criteria" air pollutants subject to national ambient air quality standards. EPA and other public health agencies continue to update the cancer risk estimates in response to new data and new scientific theories.[298]

As Gilda Radner's *Saturday Night Live* character Emily Litella would say after realizing that she had no idea what she was talking about, "Never mind."

Here's another example of the importance of looking at the actual studies. On March 9, 1999, Dan Rather reported:

There's a major study out tonight in the *Journal of the American Medical Association* contradicting a long-held belief about diet and cancer. This

14-year Harvard study of almost 89,000 women found no evidence a high-fat diet increases a woman's breast cancer risk, or that a low-fat diet cuts the risk.[299]

But 11 days later, CNN's medical correspondent Dr. Steve Salvatore reported, "In this week's *Journal of the National Cancer Institute*, researchers from the University of Southern California Medical School say cutting fat calories can reduce your risk of breast cancer." Confused? How could you not be? How is a layman supposed to interpret conflicting messages from two major medical journals within two weeks of each other? It's easier than you might think.

All you would have needed to do was read even a summary of the *Journal of the National Cancer Institute* study, which concluded, "Dietary fat reduction can result in a lowering of serum estradiol levels."[300] The study reported only that reducing dietary fat levels reduced blood levels of estradiol (an estrogen)—not the risk of breast cancer. The researchers didn't examine a possible association between dietary fat and breast cancer rates. While some studies report an increase in breast cancer rates with increased serum estradiol levels, a cause-and-effect relationship is far from proven.[301]

So the studies weren't contradictory—once you got beyond the media muddle.

Rule: Editorials Can Be Educational

Scientific and medical journals often accompany newsworthy studies with editorials that interpret the results. Sometimes the editorials are quite critical of the studies—so much so that you wonder why the journal even bothered to publish the study.

Smokers' Sons More Violent, Study Says

declared the *Los Angeles Times*, citing research published in a psychiatric journal. The news article continued:

Male children born to women who smoke during pregnancy run a risk of violent and criminal behavior that lasts well into adulthood, perhaps because of central nervous system damage, a study said. The finding was consistent with earlier studies that linked prenatal smoking not only to lawbreaking by the offspring but to impulsive behavior and attention deficit problems, said researchers at Emory University in Atlanta, USC and the Institute of Preventive Medicine in Denmark. But they said their study—based on a look at the arrest histories up to age 34 of 4,169 males born between 1959 and 1961 in Copenhagen—was the first to show that the effect lasted beyond adolescence into adulthood. The study said the mechanism behind the effect might be damage done by smoking to the central nervous system of the fetus.[302]

What the *Times* failed to mention was the accompanying editorial that stated:

The finding of consistent linkages between smoking during pregnancy and antisocial behaviors is intriguing, and these results invite the hypothesis that maternal smoking during pregnancy increases children's risk of later antisocial behavior. However, the uncertainties in these areas are such that it would be premature to conclude that maternal prenatal smoking can now be included among the established risk factors for later antisocial behaviors. There is further work to be conducted into underlying mechanisms and the possible confounding effects of genetic factors. . . . Given the ambiguities in the evidence noted above, perhaps the most prudent summation of research in this area is that maternal prenatal smoking may affect longer-term behavioral development, but considerable uncertainty still exists about the origins of the relationship.[303]

A balanced report would have mentioned the editorial to provide critical perspective on the story. But that would have made the article much less intriguing.

Rule: Watch the Quotable Quacks

Health news stories often feature quotes from "experts." The advantages of using such quotes run two ways—and neither way benefits you.

For the journalist, quotes from experts lend gravitas—or at least the appearance of it—to the report. The expert, in turn, gets desirable visibility, as quotes are generally presented in a light highly favorable to the expert. Because of that, the reporter may be somewhat less than candid in identifying the scientist.

When the news broke in June 2000 that the U.S. Environmental Protection Agency was about to restrict use of the popular insecticide Dursban, media reports were full of quotes and recommendations from Dr. Philip Landrigan:

- "If EPA does the right thing [by restricting Dursban], then it shows that they are serious about enforcing the law and serious about protecting children."[304]
- "[Dursban] is a lot like low-level lead poisoning. Children appear to be normal. It's only when you test them, that you find that they're lacking five or six or 10 points of IQ."[305]
- "And for residents trying to repel bugs, one physician, Dr. Philip Landrigan, recommended using a less-toxic product."[306]

These reports identified Landrigan as "chairman of the Department of Community and Preventive Medicine at Mount Sinai School of Medicine in New York City" or just as a "physician." Both designations were accurate—sort of.

But each report omitted mention that Landrigan is also a notorious anti-pesticide activist—an inconvenient fact that might adversely affect his credibility, don't you think?

Rule: Get the Big Picture

In their rush to scare you with a new study, journalists often fail to report how the study fits in with past research. In March 1999, CBS News health reporter David Hnida reported on *CBS This Morning*:

Most pregnant women will do all they can to make sure that their baby is born healthy and strong. They rest more, eat better and make other lifestyle changes. But very few think to take a look at their work environment as a possible hazard. But a new study in this week's *Journal of the American Medical Association* shows that pregnant women who work with organic solvents like paint thinners and industrial glues may be more likely to give birth to babies with birth defects. Researchers followed 250 pregnant women. Half worked around organic solvents, half did not. The end result: Those who worked around these chemicals had a higher rate of miscarriages, premature labor and fetal distress during labor.[307]

Hnida was referring to a study that reported, "Significantly more major malformations occurred among fetuses of women exposed to organic solvents than controls (13 vs 1; relative risk, 13.0; 95% confidence interval, 1.8–99.5)."[308]

The study has many problems, including statistical flakiness— the confidence interval is six times larger than the reported effect; there was no measurement of actual exposures to solvents; there were no clinical evaluations that the birth defects were caused by chemical exposures; and other risk factors for miscarriage weren't considered. But perhaps the biggest problem with Hnida's report was omitting the "big picture."

There are more than 550 studies in the scientific literature on exposure to chemicals and miscarriage and birth defects. Still, "Evidence of fetal damage or demise from occupational organic solvent levels that are not toxic to the pregnant woman is inconsistent in the medical literature."[309]

I'm confident it never occurred to Hnida to do a little background research on occupational exposure to organic solvents—otherwise why would he have reported so confidently on a question that so many other studies couldn't answer?

LESSON 12:
KNOW YOUR FRIENDS

*The best time to make friends is before you
need them.*

—Ethel Barrymore

WE STARTED OUT WITH the "Know Thine Enemies" lesson. We'll finish with its complement. Knowing your friends gives you a compendium of sources of useful information when health scares hit. The sources listed here are reliable and active foes of junk science. When a health scare hits, they'll often have something to say. There is no guarantee they will always be 100 percent correct. I don't always agree with them and they don't always agree with me. But I value and trust them all. You should, too.

The people, organizations, and Web sites below are usually pretty quick to comment on emerging health scares. They're your best bet when time is of the essence.

The **American Council on Science and Health** is a consumer education consortium concerned with issues related to food, nutrition, chemicals, pharmaceuticals, lifestyle, the environment, and health. ACSH is an independent, nonprofit, tax-exempt organization. The nucleus of ACSH is a board of 350 physicians, scientists, and policy advisers—experts in a wide variety of fields—who review the council's reports and participate in ACSH seminars, press conferences, media communications, and other educational activities. Classic ACSH publications include *Facts versus Fears: A Review of the Greatest Unfounded Health Scares of Recent Times* and *The Holiday Dinner Menu*. ACSH is on the Web at www.acsh.org.

The **Competitive Enterprise Institute** is a nonprofit think tank dedicated to advancing the principles of free enterprise and limited government. CEI issue areas include air pollution, biotechnology and food regulation, drug and medical device regulation, tobacco and smoking, chemical and environmental risk, global warming, and environmental education. CEI is on the Web at www.cei.org.

Michael Fumento is an author, journalist, and attorney specializing in science and health issues with the Hudson Institute. He has been a legal writer for the *Washington Times* and an editorial writer for the *Rocky Mountain News* in Denver. He was the first "National Issues" reporter for *Investor's Business Daily*. You'll see Mr. Fumento's articles in many magazines, including *Reader's Digest*, the *Atlantic Monthly*, *Forbes*, the *New Republic*, *USA Weekend*, the *Washington Monthly*, *Reason*, the *Weekly Standard*, *National Review*, *Policy Review*, and the *American Spectator*. Mr. Fumento has published in such newspapers as the *Wall Street Journal*, the *New York Times*, the *Washington Post*, the *Christian Science Monitor*, the *Sunday Times* (London), the *Sunday Telegraph* (London), the *Los Angeles Times*, *Investor's Business Daily*, the *Washington Times*, and the *Chicago Tribune*. Fumento's Web site is www.fumento.com.

Dr. Michael Gough is an adjunct scholar at the Cato Institute. Dr. Gough directed the now-defunct Congressional Office of Technology Assessment's oversight of executive branch studies of cancer in veterans of atomic bomb tests and of the health of Vietnam veterans. He chaired a Department of Veterans' Affairs advisory committee (1987–90) on the health effects of herbicides used in Vietnam and the Department of Health and Human Services advisory committee (1990–95) for the U.S. Air Force study of the health of Air Force personnel who sprayed Agent Orange in Vietnam. In 1995 he was a government expert on the U.S. Environmental Protection Agency's Science Advisory Board committee that evaluated EPA's dioxin reassessment. Gough has published two dozen papers in molecular biology, genetics, and microbiology. He is the author of *Dioxin, Agent Orange*; coeditor, with T. S. Glickman, of *Readings in Risk*; coauthor, with Steven J. Milloy, of *Silencing Science*; and author of more than 40 papers about environmental and occupational health as well as numerous newspaper op-eds. He has testified about three dozen times before Congress. He is a fellow of the Society for Risk Analysis and vice-president of the International Society for Regulatory Toxicology and Pharmacology (1999–2001). The Cato Institute's Web site is www.cato.org.

Dr. Henry I. Miller is a senior research fellow at the Hoover Institution. His research focuses on science and technology and their regulation; pharmaceutical development and regulation; and federal, domestic, and international oversight of the products of genetic engineering. Dr. Miller joined the U.S. Food and Drug Administration in 1979 and served in a number of posts involved with the new biotechnology. He was the medical reviewer for the first genetically engineered drugs evaluated by the FDA and was instrumental in the rapid licensing of human insulin and human growth hormone. He served in several posts, including special assistant to the FDA commissioner, with responsibility for biotechnology issues; and in 1989–94 he was the founding director of the FDA's Office of Biotechnology. His monographs include "Policy Controversy in Biotechnology: An Insider's View," "Biotechnology Regulation: The Unacceptable Costs of Excessive Regulation," and "To America's Health: A Model for Reform of the Food and Drug Administration." In addition, he has published extensively in prominent medical, scientific, and public affairs journals and newspapers worldwide, including the *Lancet*, *Journal of the American Medical Association*, *Science*, *Nature*, *Nature Biotech-*

nology, the *Weekly Standard*, the *National Review*, the *Wall Street Journal*, the *New York Times*, and the *Financial Times*. The Hoover Institution is online at www.hoover.org.

NutritionNewsFocus.com e-mails free, succinct analyses of the latest nutrition issues. Most of the material is provided by Dr. David Klurfeld, the head of the Department of Nutrition and Food Sciences at Wayne State University. This newsletter provides reliable information. Each e-mail ends with a "WHAT YOU NEED TO KNOW" blurb. NNF is on the Web at www.nutritionnewsfocus.com.

Quackwatch.com, a member of Consumer Federation of America, is a nonprofit corporation whose purpose is to combat health-related frauds, myths, fads, and fallacies. Activities include investigating questionable claims, answering inquiries, distributing reliable publications, reporting illegal marketing, generating consumer protection lawsuits, improving the quality of health information on the Internet, and attacking misleading advertising on the Internet. The Web site is www.quackwatch.com.

Sally Satel is a lecturer at the Yale University School of Medicine, staff psychiatrist at the Oasis Clinic, Washington, D.C., and an adjunct scholar at the American Enterprise Institute. In addition to numerous scientific publications, Dr. Satel's articles and opinion pieces have appeared in the *Wall Street Journal*, the *New York Times*, the *New Republic*, *National Review*, *Public Interest*, the *Los Angeles Times*, *City Journal* (of the Manhattan Institute), and *SLATE*. Dr. Satel is also the author of *PC M.D.—How Political Correctness Is Corrupting Medicine*.

The **Statistical Assessment Service** examines the way that scientific, quantitative, and social research are presented by the media and works with journalists to help them convey this material accurately and effectively. STATS sponsors the annual Dubious Data Awards and has a monthly publication called *VitalSTATS*. STATS is on the Web at www.stats.org.

And of course, don't forget www.JunkScience.com.

That's it, you ask? There's no one else to turn to? Sure, there are lots of other experts who are knowledgeable about the issues involved in health scares. But the people, organizations, and Web sites named here are the "go to" resources dedicated to helping set the scientific record straight. They're the always-prepared, no-holds-barred pros that I recommend.

A FINAL WORD: GO FORTH AND DEBUNK

We shall fight on the beaches, we shall fight on the landing grounds, we shall fight in the fields and in the streets; we shall fight in the hills; we shall never surrender.

—Winston Churchill

I TRUST THAT YOU have been attentive and by now have earned your "black belt" in Junk Science Judo. You'll certainly find use for it in a world where health research often has more in common with professional wrestling than with science. There is no free lunch, however—and I'm not referring just to the cost of this book.

If you're familiar with the martial arts, you know that with advanced skills comes an obligation to teach—to pass on the message. Your Junk Science Judo black belt confers a similar moral obligation to fight the junk science machine. The people who profit from promoting junk science are highly motivated. They are organized and often well financed. But don't for a minute be discouraged. You know their weaknesses. I hope you live up to your new civic responsibility. Here are some ways to carry on the fight.

Provide Feedback

Gripe to the News Media

File complaints with broadcasters and publishers when you hear or see junk science–filled news reports. You never know when you'll strike a nerve. You never know whether someone inside the offending news organization has raised the same objections. Your voice will strengthen the unknown friend. But if you don't complain, media types may never know they got the story wrong. If lots of people like you and me speak up, they will get the message.

Send letters to newspapers. Telephone radio and television stations. E-mail Internet sites. Make your complaint crisp and pointed—no more than a couple hundred words, if written. Don't rant and rave. Get your facts and citations straight. Spotlight precisely what was scientifically wrong with the report at issue. Be ready to send more detailed information if requested. Follow up. Send your complaint to the editor or producer and send a copy to the reporter.

Encourage friends and colleagues to echo your complaint. Your goal should be to get your views published or aired. Then others will learn from you. If you get an apology or retraction—don't hold your breath—you've hit a home run. Complaining may not completely undo the damage done by the original report, but it's better than doing nothing. You'd be surprised at the number of readers who turn to the "Letters" column of their daily paper with their morning coffee. You *can* make a difference.

Gripe to Elected Officials

Federal, state, and local governments often take action on the basis of junk science. Alert your elected representatives to junk science problems. They're unlikely to notice or take action on their own. Get others to do the same. Request a meeting to explain your views. Get others to support your efforts.

Gripe to Businesses That Use Junk Science

Reputable businesses shouldn't be making health claims that can't be backed up with *real* scientific evidence. Let them know that. Support businesses that are attacked with junk science. An unfortunate reaction by businesses attacked with junk science is to reformulate their products; they think it's smarter to switch than fight. That's a shortsighted tactic, though. Any sort of validation of junk science simply spawns subsequent junk science–fueled attacks.

It's often against the nature of levelheaded people to become activists. That's one reason the junk science mobsters have been so successful. They don't think twice about activism. They're so aggressive that they appear to be unopposed. Don't be fooled. In fact, there is much opposition to the perversion of science. Too often, though, that opposition simmers quietly rather than steams publicly. So blow your top!

Advocate Anti–Junk Science Public Policy

Governments generate a lot of junk science. Here are some ways to reduce junk science by changing public policy.

Separate Researchers and Regulators

We hear a lot about how academic research is "corrupted" by private industry funding. In the immortal words of ABC News's John Stossel, "Give me a break!" Politicians and bureaucrats pushing personal crusades and biased agendas are not above misrepresenting scientific "evidence" to advance a favored policy.

Regulatory agencies fund and conduct studies, evaluate the results, and then decide how to regulate on the basis of their "science." They're judge, jury, and executioner, all in one convenient package. This system allows agencies to cook up science as needed to achieve predetermined outcomes. On the basis of junk science, agencies promulgate regulations with the force of law. Because courts are reluctant to intervene and often barred from doing so, the public usually has no legal recourse against government agencies. As in Inquisition days, dogma, not reason, rules the roost.

Research should be designed, conducted, and reviewed by scientists totally independent of the regulatory agencies. Tell your congresspersons to insist on a firewall between researchers and regulators.

Require Public Access to Data

The scientific method calls for replication of study results by independent researchers. This is easy enough with laboratory studies; all researchers need do is disclose their materials and methods. For epidemiologic studies, in contrast, replication efforts require access to the original data—and therein lies the rub.

Epidemiologists are reluctant to provide their raw data to other researchers. Now that you understand how flaky epidemiology can be, you can understand their reluctance—which can become downright defiance.

The Environmental Protection Agency proposed in November 1996 more stringent regulation of airborne fine particulate matter (PM). The EPA initially claimed further regulation would prevent 20,000 "premature deaths." But the EPA's estimate was quite controversial. You'll remember that it depended on a single ecologic-type study reporting a weak statistical association. When the controversy prompted Congress to ask the EPA to produce the study's raw data for independent analysis, the EPA balked, saying there was no purpose in any re-analysis of the EPA-funded study. Eventually, but only *after* the EPA issued the regulations, access to the study data was given to a single research organization. That was not a victory for scientific openness and review. The organization chosen to review the findings receives one-half of its funding from the EPA.

Because of difficulty in obtaining the study data, a federal law was enacted in October 1998 requiring that federally funded scientific data used to support federal policy must be publicly available through the Freedom of Information Act.

Since the law's enactment, the junk science mobsters have fought to have the law repealed. They don't want to be scrutinized by the public. But scrutiny is part of science.

Insist on Adequate Judicial Review

Government agencies use junk science with virtual impunity. In court, decisions of federal regulatory agencies are usually adjudged by the very loose standard of "arbitrary and capricious," contained in the Administrative Procedures Act.[310]

To meet the "arbitrary and capricious" standard, an agency needs to present only a bare bones rationale for taking action. As long as a rationale is presented—including the most egregious junk science—courts are reluctant to second-guess the agency.[311] Agencies are assumed to be experts in their areas of regulation.

Of course, you should be so lucky as to get an agency into court in the first place. Few laws allow federal agencies to be challenged on the basis of faulty science. In contrast, many laws—especially environmental laws—allow the Junksters easy access to courts to challenge agencies.

To check regulatory agency use of junk science, the public should be allowed greater leeway to challenge agencies in court. Agencies should be required to defend their actions on the basis of a standard of, at least, "substantial evidence."

The U.S. Occupational Safety and Health Administration (OSHA) is required to justify its actions on the basis of "substantial evidence." This evidentiary standard has been a major barrier to OSHA's use of junk science in the setting of worker safety standards. In 1992, for example, a federal court struck down OSHA's permissible exposure limits (PELs) for 428 substances on the basis that assumptions used by OSHA in the risk assessments supporting the PELs were not substantiated by the available scientific evidence.[312] The court said that while assumptions may be used in risk assessment, they must have some basis in fact.

Congress should change the Administrative Procedures Act to apply the "substantial evidence" standard to all regulatory bodies. That would be a start.

Support Daubert Panels

There is a significant impediment to personal injury lawyers running amok in the federal courtrooms. Federal trial judges may convene so-called Daubert panels—groups of experts selected by courts to review scientific or other technical evidence before trial.

The purpose of a Daubert panel is to keep junk science out of the courtroom by helping the judge determine what scientific facts and testimony should be admitted as evidence. A federal judge must "ensure that any and all scientific testimony or evidence admitted is not only relevant, but reliable," according to the Supreme Court.[313]

How successful have Daubert panels been? Since 1974, in 73 federal lawsuits involving product liability and toxic tort in which the plaintiff has sought to admit expert testimony about cause-and-effect relationships, the district courts admitted only 23 experts.[314] Similarly, the federal appellate courts allowed only 10 of 31 experts to testify on causation.

But not all state courts use Daubert panels. Even where Daubert panels are allowed, judges can skirt them. While there's no way to ensure that judges make correct decisions when faced with scientific questions, they should at least have the opportunity to enlist expert assistance.

Make sure your state allows judges to convene Daubert panels.

Be Prepared, Chicago-Style

Make no mistake. If you criticize the Junksters, you open yourself up to attack by them. Certainly their best and most likely strategy is to ignore critics. Responding to your criticism may prolong and spotlight a debate they know they can't win. They're betting that you'll go away because you have better things to do. (They don't. Junk science is their livelihood.)

If you persist and especially if you succeed, prepare yourself for savage retaliation. It will almost certainly follow. I've been viciously attacked through media releases, Web sites, and even a book. I've been threatened with lawsuits. The most prominent environmental groups wrote a letter demanding that the Cato Institute disassociate itself from me. The Society of Environmental Journalists once invited me to speak on a panel where I was to be ambushed by the other panelists.

The Junksters' chief tactic is to shoot the messenger when they don't like the message. If you criticize the Junksters, then they say you are doing so only because you're in the pockets of their opponents. Even if that were true, so what?

In response to an article in *Science* reporting that tobacco industry consultants were compensated for writing letters to science journals, I responded:

> [The] article "Tobacco consultants find letters lucrative" (News of the Week, 14 Aug., p. 895) presents only one side of the funding story. The anti-tobacco industry pays its scientists, too.
>
> The U.S. Occupational Safety and Health Administration (OSHA) paid University of California (San Francisco) anti-tobacco activist Stanton Glantz $25,000 to testify at the 1994 OSHA hearings on indoor air quality and to summarize the hearings. All told, OSHA paid $150,000 for scientists to testify in favor of its proposal. The National Cancer Institute paid Glantz over $600,000 to research tobacco industry lobbying. Backup documentation is available on both counts.
>
> Meanwhile, Glantz "fumes" because the tobacco industry paid scientists to write letters? The funding story cuts both ways. You can't cover one side without covering the other. The $150,000 spent by the tobacco industry pales in comparison to the hundreds of millions (billions?) of dollars that go into federal and state anti-tobacco programs. And while we are talking about funding, how about the $2 billion in federal money that goes to scientists supporting the Clinton Administration on global warming? That is a lot more than the global warming skeptics receive from industry.

> We are better off focusing on the merits of scientific arguments, not who pays to broadcast them, lest we fall into the trap of shooting the messenger because we do not like the message.

The Junksters fear science and desperately need to change the subject. Ad hominem attacks turn the facts into a side issue. Stay on the science, but be prepared to fight back, Chicago-style.

Remember these lines uttered by Sean Connery to Kevin Costner as Eliot Ness in the movie *The Untouchables*: "He pulls a knife on you, you pull a gun. He sends one of yours to the hospital, you send one of his to the morgue. That's the Chicago way."

Be Undaunted by Junk Science Tyranny

Junk science has always existed—alchemy, astrology, and haruspicy were a few of its early forms. It won't disappear soon, if ever. There probably always will be dishonest characters who, under the guise of "science," try to deceive others with bogus data and analysis.

At present, the junk science mob is well entrenched in our society, having established itself in the highest levels of the scientific community and the government. The mob is a formidable force. Fighting it can be akin to beating your head against a wall. It is painful and frustrating. That's guaranteed. So remember the immortal words of Thomas Paine in his December 1776 pamphlet, *The Crisis*:

> These are the times that try men's souls. The summer soldier and the sunshine patriot will, in this crisis, shrink from the service of their country; but he that stands it now, deserves the love and thanks of man and woman. Tyranny, like hell, is not easily conquered; yet we have this consolation with us, that the harder the conflict, the more glorious the triumph. What we obtain too cheap, we esteem too lightly: it is dearness only that gives every thing its value.

A December 25, 1776, reading of *The Crisis* inspired George Washington's ragtag army as it crossed the Delaware River to launch a surprise attack and defeat the British and Hessian mercenaries encamped at Trenton, New Jersey, on December 26, 1776.

If those words could inspire demoralized, hungry troops with rags for shoes to mount an attack in freezing winter weather, they should suffice as encouragement for you, the newly minted junk science judoist.

NOTES

Preface

1. See K. J. Cruickshanks, R. Klein, B. E. Klein, T. L. Wiley, D. M. Nondahl, T. S. Tweed, "Cigarette Smoking and Hearing Loss: The Epidemiology of Hearing Loss Study," *Journal of the American Medical Association,* June 3, 1998, pp. 1715–19.

2. P. Cummings, D. C. Grossman, F. P. Rivara, T. D. Koepsell, "State Gun Safe Storage Laws and Child Mortality due to Firearms," *Journal of the American Medical Association,* October 1, 1997, pp. 1084–86.

3. E. R. Shell. "The Hippocratic Wars," *New York Times Magazine,* June 28, 1998.

4. S. A. Sanders, J. M. Reinisch, "Would You Say You 'Had Sex' If . . . ?" *Journal of the American Medical Association*, January 20, 1999, pp. 275–77.

5. Statement of AMA executive vice president E. Ratcliffe Anderson, Jr., M.D., January 15, 1999.

Introduction

6. B. Mittler, "Media Often Mislead Public on Health Issues," *Tulsa World*, April 7, 1999.

7. B. Mittler, "Anatomy of a Media Drug Scare," *Wall Street Journal*, August 2, 1996.

8. See, for example, *Nature*, November 28, 1991.

9. U.S. Centers for Disease Control and Prevention, "Ten Great Public Health Achievements—United States, 1900-1999," *Morbidity and Mortality Weekly Report*, April 2, 1999, pp. 241–43.

10. D. R. Roberts, L. L. Laughlin, P. Hsheih, L. J. Legters, "DDT, Global Strategies, and a Malaria Control Crisis in South America," *Emerging Infectious Diseases*, July–September, 1997, pp. 295–302.

11. R. A. Kronmal, C. W. Whitney, S. D. Mumford, "The Intrauterine Device and Pelvic Inflammatory Disease: The Women's Health Study Reanalyzed," *Journal of Clinical Epidemiology*, February 1991, pp. 109–22.

12. J. Concato, "Prostate Specific Antigen: A Useful Screening Test?" *Cancer Journal from Scientific American*, April 6, 2000, pp. S188–92.

13. "Prostate Blood Test in Development," *Cancer Weekly Plus*, May 17, 1999.

14. S. J. Milloy, "The Tail End of the Fiber Myth," October 13, 2000, http://www.foxnews.com/science/JunkScience/001013.sml (October 13, 2000).

15. http://www.floridajuice.com/floridacitrus/health.htm#heart.

16. See, for example, S. Liu, J. E. Manson, I. M. Lee, S. R. Cole, C. H. Hennekens, W. C. Willett, J. E. Buring, "Fruit and Vegetable Intake and Risk of Cardiovascular Disease: The Women's Health Study," *American Journal of Clinical Nutrition*, October 2000, pp. 922–28.

17. "Problematic Partnership, Heart Association 'Certifications' Undermine Charity's Credibility, Critics Say," *Chicago Tribune*, November 5, 1997.

18. B. M. Rifkind, J. E. Rossouw, "Of Designer Drugs, Magic Bullets, and Gold Standards," *Journal of the American Medical Association*, May 13, 1998, pp. 1483–85.

19. See, for example, "Greener Greens? The Truth about Organic Food," *Consumer Reports*, January 1998.

20. U.S. Department of Agriculture. Economic Research Service. Food Cost Review, 1950–97, http://www.ers.usda.gov.

21. "Radon Blamed for 18,000 Lung-Cancer Deaths in U.S. Each Year," *Washington Post*, February 20, 1998.

22. See, for example, "Study Finds Radioactive Particles May Be More Damaging Than Expected," Associated Press, April 26, 1999.

23. "Woman Removes Own Breast Implants with Razorblade," Agence France Presse, April 17, 1992.

24. E. M. Whelan, "A Morbid Fear of Illness Makes America Trash Good Food and Common Sense," *Los Angeles Times*, March 10, 1989.

25. "A President with No Shame," *Denver Post*, December 22, 1995.

26. "Shutdown Threatens Cleanup of Toxic Waste Sites, EPA Warns," *Los Angeles Times*, December 30, 1995.

Lesson 1

27. NRDC's Washington, D.C., communications director Eliot Negin quoted in *Inside PR*, September 4, 2000.

28. "Apple Industry Issues Response to '60 Minutes' Broadcast," PR Newswire, March 1, 1989, www.prnewswire.com.

29. ABC News, "Mayo Clinic Issues Urgent Warning on Fen-phen," *World News Tonight*, July 8, 1997.

30. The two drugs were fenfluramine and phentermine.

31. "New Context; Statistical Data Included," *ADWEEK*, May 29, 2000, eastern edition.

32. The conference was the 20th International Symposium on Halogenated Environmental Organic Pollutants & POPS, August 13–17, 2000.

33. "Vinyl IV Bags May Leach Liver-damaging Toxins," *Boston Herald*, February 22, 1999.

34. "Blood Bags Deemed Dangerous," *Calgary Herald*, February 23, 1999.

35. "Groups Assert IV Bags Pose Dangers to Multiple Organs," *Chicago Tribune*, June 21, 1999.

36. "Environmental Groups Report Chemicals Added to IV Bags Are Leaching into Patients' Blood and May Be Dangerous," National Public Radio, *All Things Considered*, February 22, 1999.

37. "Doctors Asked by Environmental Groups to Stop Using IV Bags Made of PVC Plastic," CBS News, February 22, 1999.

38. "Agency Takes DEHP Off Carcinogen List," *Plastics News*, March 7, 2000.

39. S. J. Milloy, "Media Lose Message," *Chicago Sun Times*, March 27, 2000.

40. There is even a new school of thought among journalists called "civic journalism," according to which merely reporting the news is insufficient; journalists should tailor their reports to promote political activism.

41. "Woman's Breast Implant Suit Started Dominoes Falling," *Idaho Statesman*, March 14, 1992.

42. They had not been proven unsafe either. There was simply a lack of data.

43. M. Angell, *Science on Trial: The Clash of Medical Evidence and the Law in the Breast Implant Case* (New York: W.W. Norton, 1996).

44. S. E. Gabriel, W. M. O'Fallon, L. T. Kurland, C. M. Beard, J. E. Woods, L. J. Melton III, "Risk of Connective-tissue Diseases and Other Disorders after Breast Implantation," *New England Journal of Medicine*, June 16, 1994, pp. 1697–702.

45. See, for example, E. C. Janowsky, L. L. Kupper, B. S. Hulka, "Meta-analyses of the Relation between Silicone Breast Implants and the Risk of Connective-tissue Diseases," *New England Journal of Medicine*, March 16, 2000, pp. 781–90.

46. "Lancet Publishes New Study Linking Silicone Implants to Immune Problems; Blood Test Able to Identify Women with Severe Symptoms of Atypical Disease; Adds to Growing Body of Research," PR Newswire, February 13, 1997.

47. "Research Links Breast Implants to New Disease," *Times-Picayune,* February 15, 1997.

48. Untitled, PR Newswire, February 18, 1997.

49. "Jury: Dow Hid Implant Danger; Plaintiffs Must Prove Injuries," *Times-Picayune*, August 19, 1997.

50. *Frontline*, February 27, 1996.

51. The references for this incident are at http://www.JunkScience.com/sep99/anradmit.htm.

52. See http://www.JunkScience.com/sep99/anradmit.htm.

53. Pete Hanauer, Americans for Nonsmokers Rights, e-mail to Michael Siegel, August 31, 1999.

54. American Council on Science and Health, "The Plot against Alar," *Priorities for Health*," 1991.

55. "Consumer Advocate Announces Drive against Apple Chemical," Associated Press, July 6, 1986.

56. See M. Fumento, *Science under Siege: Balancing Technology and the Environment* (New York: William Morrow, 1993) pp. 19–20.

57. B. Sewell, R. Whyatt, *Intolerable Risk: Pesticides in Our Children's Foods* (New York: Natural Resources Defense Council, February 1989).

58. "How a PR Firm Executed the Alar Scare," extracted from a Fenton Communications memorandum, *Wall Street Journal*, October 3, 1989.

59. For those of you who didn't watch television in the 1970s, Redd Foxx starred as junkyard dealer Fred Sanford in the situation comedy *Sanford & Son*.

60. V. Beral, E. Banks, G. Reeves, P. Appleby, "Use of HRT and the Subsequent Risk of Cancer," *Journal of Epidemiology and Biostatistics*, April 1999, pp. 191–215.

61. "Health and Well-being: A Way through the HRT Maze: Continuing Our Series on the Menopause, Christine Doyle Looks at Hormone Replacement Therapy," *Daily Telegraph*, February 15, 2000.

62. J. K. Dunnick, J. F. Hardisty, R. A. Herbert, J. C. Seely, E. M. Furedi-Machacek, J. F. Foley, G. C. Lacks, S. Stasiewicz, J. E. French, "Phenolphthalein Induces Thymic Lymphomas Accompanied by Loss of the p53 Wild Type Allele in Heterozygous p53-deficient (+/-) Mice," *Toxicologic Pathology*, November-December 1997, pp. 533–40.

63. "Scientists Find Ingredient in Common Laxative Causes Cancer in Rats," Associated Press, April 30, 1997.

64. See "The Experiment That Could Clobber Ex-Lax," Business Week, June 30, 1997; and "Schering's Laxative Ad Brings Negative Outburst; Schering-Plough Healthcare Products's Advertisement Which Claims That Laxatives May Cause Cancer," Medical Marketing & Media, August, 1997.

65. "The Experiment That Could Clobber Ex-Lax."

66. M. Fumento, "The Zapping of Sensormatic," Forbes, January 25, 1999.

67. "Scientist's Pacemaker Research Sparks PR Battle," St. Petersburg Times, March 14, 1999.

68. Robert O'Holla, vice president of regulatory affairs, Johnson & Johnson, Testimony at the House Commerce Oversight and Investigations Committee's inquiry into reuse of medical devices, February 10, 2000.

69. K. F. Browne, R. Maldonado, M. Telatnik, R. E. Vlietstra, A. S. Brenner, "Initial Experience with Reuse of Coronary Angioplasty Catheters in the United States," Journal of the American College of Cardiology, December 30, 1997, pp. 1735–40.

70. "FDA Exposes Patients to Risks of Medical Recycling," USA Today, November 30, 1999.

71. "These Devices Are Safe," USA Today, November 29, 1999.

72. See U.S. Department of Health and Human Services, "FDA Releases Final Guidance on the Reprocessing and Reuse of Single-use Devices," User Facility Reporting, Summer 2000.

73. R. L. Pearson, H. Wachtel, K. L. Ebi, "Distance-weighted Traffic Density in Proximity to a Home Is a Risk Factor for Leukemia and Other Childhood Cancers," Journal of the Air and Waste Management Association, February 2000, pp. 175–80.

74. J. M. Peters, S. Preston-Martin, S. J. London, J. D. Bowman, J. D. Buckley, D. C. Thomas, "Processed Meats and Risk of Childhood Leukemia," Cancer Causes and Control, March 1994, pp. 195–202.

75. National Research Council, Possible Health Effects of Exposure to Residential Electric and Magnetic Fields (Washington: National Academy Press, 1996).

76. See "Kellogg Seeks FDA Approval for Health Claim; By Asserting a Link Between Wheat Bran Intake and Reduced Risk of Colon Cancer, the Cereal Maker May Be Able to Target Its Advertising and Boost Stagnant Sales," Chicago Tribune, June 4, 1997.

77. C. S. Fuchs, E. L. Giovannucci, G. A. Colditz. D. J. Hunter, M. J. Stampfer, B. Rosner, F. E. Speizer, W. C. Willett, "Dietary Fiber and the Risk of Colorectal Cancer and Adenoma in Women," New England Journal of Medicine, January 21, 1999, pp. 169–76.

78. See D. S. Alberts, M. E. Martinez, D. J. Roe, J. M. Guillen-Rodriguez, J. R. Marshall, J. B. van Leeuwen, M. E. Reid, C. Ritenbaugh, P. A. Vargas, A. B. Bhattacharyya, D. L. Earnest, R. E. Sampliner, "Lack of Effect of a High-fiber Cereal Supplement on the Recurrence of Colorectal Adenomas," New England Journal of Medicine, April 20, 2000, pp. 1156-62; A. Schatzkin, E. Lanza, D. Corle, P. Lance, F. Iber, B. Caan, M. Shike, J. Weissfeld, R. Burt, M. R. Cooper, J. W. Kikendall, J. Cahill, Polyp Prevention Trial Study Group, "Lack of Effect of a Low-fat, High-fiber Diet on the Recurrence of Colorectal Adenomas," New England Journal of Medicine, April 20, 2000, pp. 1149-55; C. Bonithon-Kopp, O. Kronborg, A. Giacosa, U. Räth, J. Faivre, "Calcium and Fibre Supplementation in Prevention of Colorectal Adenoma Recurrence: A Randomised Intervention Trial," Lancet, October 14, 2000, pp. 1300–306.

79. American Council on Science and Health, "Science Panel Rejects Kellogg's Claims That Cereal Prevents Colon Cancer," August 28, 1998.

80. "Dangerous Cardiovascular Effect of Second Hand Smoke May Be Reduced by Drinking Purple Grape Juice," PR Newswire, April 19, 1999.

81. Ibid.

82. See, for example, "Greener Greens? The Truth about Organic Food," *Consumer Reports*, January 1998.

83. R. C. Miller, G. Randers-Pehrson, C. R. Geard, E. J. Hall, D. J. Brenner, "The Oncogenic Transforming Potential of the Passage of Single Alpha Particles through Mammalian Cell Nuclei," *Proceedings of the National Academy of Sciences*, January 5, 1999, pp. 19–22.

84. "Clinton Extending Agent Orange Coverage," Associated Press, May 28, 1996.

85. "A Bad Agent Orange Decision," editorial, *Washington Post*, May 31, 1996.

86. "Clinton Camp Is Splintered on Next Step," *Washington Post*, August 20, 1998.

87. B. Hileman, "Fluoridation of Water," *Chemical Engineering News*, August 1, 1988, pp. 26–42.

88. This Cold War paranoia was even reflected in the movie *Dr. Strangelove: Or How I Learned to Stop Worrying and Love the Bomb*. General Jack D. Ripper (played by Peter Sellers) said, "I can no longer sit back and allow Communist infiltration, Communist indoctrination, Communist subversion and the international Communist conspiracy to sap and impurify all of our precious bodily fluids."

89. See National Toxicology Program, *Toxicology and Carcinogenesis Studies of Sodium Fluoride in F344/N Rats and B6C3F₁ Mice*, Technical Report Series 393, NIH Publication no. 91-2848 (Research Triangle Park, N.C.: National Institute of Environmental Health Sciences, 1990).

90. U.S. Environmental Protection Agency, http://www.epa.gov/pesticides/op/malathion.htm.

91. "Study Finds Food Supply in Jeopardy; Regulatory System Fails to Catch Contamination," *Orange County Register*, January 12, 1987.

92. W. E. Garthright, D. L. Archer, J. E. Kvenberg, "Estimates of Incidence and Costs of Intestinal Infectious Diseases in the United States," *Public Health Report*, March-April 1988, pp. 107–15.

93. See Angell, *Science on Trial*.

94. M. Angell, "Shattuck Lecture—Evaluating the Health Risks of Breast Implants: The Interplay of Medical Science, the Law, and Public Opinion," *New England Journal of Medicine*, June 6, 1996, pp. 1513–18.

95. P. D. Fey, T. J. Safranek, M. E. Rupp, E. F. Dunne, E. Ribot, P. C. Iwen, P. A. Bradford, F. J. Angulo, S. H. Hinrichs, "Ceftriaxone-resistant Salmonella Infection Acquired by a Child from Cattle," *New England Journal of Medicine*, April 27, 2000, pp. 1242–49.

96. "Boy's Drug-Resistant Germ Tied to Antibiotics in Cattle," *Washington Post*, April 27, 2000.

97. Centers for Disease Control and Prevention, *1999 Annual Report: National Antimicrobial Resistance Monitoring System*.

98. M. T. Osterholm, "Emerging Infections—Another Warning," *New England Journal of Medicine*, April 27, 2000, pp. 1280–81.

99. Quoted in Angell, "Shattuck Lecture."

100. "Hippocratic Wars," *New York Times Magazine*, June 28, 1998.

101. Royal Society of Canada, *A Review of the Potential Health Risks of Radiofrequency Fields from Wireless Telecommunications Devices*, May 1999, http://www.rsc.ca/english/RFreport.pdf.

102. Independent Expert Group on Mobile Phones, *Mobile Phones and Health: A Report from the Independent Expert Group on Mobile Phones*, April 2000, http://www.iegmp.org.uk/IEGMPp11.htm.

103. "'Positive Results' in WTR Brain Tumor Epi Study," *Microwave News*, March-April 1999.

104. "Angelos' Decision to File Wireless Lawsuit Expected Soon," *Radio Communications Report*, June 5, 2000.

Lesson 2

105. F. Bacon, *Novum Organum*, Book 2.

106. "Mind Over Matter," *Los Angeles Times*, December 24, 1998.

107. R. Descartes, *Discourse on Method*, part 2.

108. R. Moscati, D. Jehle, D. Ellis, A. Fiorello, M. Landi, "Positive-outcome Bias: Comparison of Emergency Medicine and General Medicine Literatures," *Academy of Emergency Medicine*, May–June 1994, pp. 267–71.

109. A. Thornton, P. Lee, "Publication Bias in Meta-analysis: Its Causes and Consequences," *Journal of Clinical Epidemiology*, February 2000, pp. 207–16.

110. "Hippocratic Wars," *New York Times Magazine*, June 28, 1998.

111. J. Swales, "Population Advice on Salt Restriction: The Social Issues," *American Journal of Hypertension*, January 13, 2001, pp. 2–7.

112. Ibid.

113. U.S. Environmental Protection Agency, *Respiratory Health Effects of Passive Smoking: Lung Cancer and Other Disorders*, December 1992.

114. See *Flue-cured Tobacco Cooperative Stabilization Corporation, the Council for Burley Tobacco, Inc., Universal Leaf Tobacco Company, Incorporated, Philip Morris Incorporated, RJ Reynolds Tobacco Company, and Gallins Vending Company v. United States Environmental Protection Agency*, 6:93CV00370, July 17, 1998 (U.S. District Court for the Middle District of North Carolina Winston-Salem Division).

115. "Could Too Much Cleanliness Make People Sick?" CNN, *Talk Back Live*, July 19, 2000.

116. Levy's theory is called the "hygiene hypothesis."

117. S. Kaplan, J. Morris, "Kids at Risk," *U.S. News and World Report*, June 19, 2000.

118. R. D. Kimbrough, R. A. Squire, R. E. Linder, J. D. Strandberg, R. J. Montalli, V. W. Burse, "Induction of Liver Tumor in Sherman Strain Female Rats by Polychlorinated Biphenyl Aroclor 1260," *Journal of the National Cancer Institute*, December 1995, pp. 1453–59.

119. R. D. Kimbrough, M. L. Doemland, M. E. LeVois, "Mortality in Male and Female Capacitor Workers Exposed to Polychlorinated Biphenyls," *Journal of Occupational and Environmental Medicine*, March 1999, pp. 161–71.

120. See, for example, J. L. Jacobson, S. W. Jacobson, "Evidence for PCBs as Neurodevelopmental Toxicants in Humans," *Neurotoxicology*, 1997, pp. 415–24 (review); J. L Jacobson, S. W. Jacobson. "Intellectual Impairment in Children Exposed to Polychlorinated Biphenyls in Utero," *New England Journal of Medicine*, September 1996, pp. 783–89; J. L. Jacobson, S. W. Jacobson, "Dose-response in Perinatal Exposure to Polychlorinated Biphenyls (PCBs): The Michigan and North Carolina Cohort Studies," *Toxicology and Industrial Health*, May–August 1996, pp. 435–45.

121. "Dioxin Is Found to be Present in Mothers' Milk," *Chemical Week*, January 20, 1988.

122. "Incinerator Gets Bath, Dioxins Drop," *Tampa Tribune*, January 9, 1996.

123. "Tampon Trashing," (New York) *Daily News*, February 6, 1997.

124. H. M. Connolly, J. L. Crary, M. D. McGoon, D. D. Hensrud, B. S. Edwards, W. D. Edwards, H. V. Schaff, "Valvular Heart Disease Associated with Fenfluramine-phentermine," *New England Journal of Medicine*, August 28, 1997, pp. 581–88.

125. See A. H. Mokdad, M. K. Serdula, W. H Dietz, B. A. Bowman, J. S. Marks, J. P. Koplan, "The Continuing Epidemic of Obesity in the United States," *Journal of the American Medical Association*, October 4, 2000, pp. 1650–51.

126. Adapted from Regulatory Impact Analysis Project, *Choices in Risk Assessment: The Role of Science Policy in the Environmental Risk Management Process*, Washington, 1994.

127. U.S. Environmental Protection Agency, "Interim Procedures and Guidelines for Health Risks and Economic Impacts of Suspected Carcinogens," *Federal Regulation,* 1976, pp. 21,402–05.

128. J. M. Peters, S. Preston-Martin, S. J. London, J. D. Bowman, J. D. Buckley, D. C. Thomas, "Processed Meats and Risk of Childhood Leukemia," *Cancer Causes and Control,* March 5, 1994, pp. 195–202.

129. Ibid.

130. .See L. H. Kushi, A. R. Folsom, R. J. Prineas, P. J. Mink, Y. Wu, R. M. Bostick, "Dietary Antioxidant Vitamins and Death from Coronary Heart Disease in Postmenopausal Women," *New England Journal of Medicine*, May 2, 1996, pp. 1156–62.

131. See J. M. Samet, F. Dominici, F. C. Curriero, I. Coursac, S. L. Zeger, "Fine Particulate Air Pollution and Mortality in 20 U.S. Cities, 1987–1994," *New England Journal of Medicine*, December 14, 2000, pp. 1742–49.

132. S. F. Arnold, D. M. Klotz, B. M. Collins, P. M. Vonier, L. J. Guillette Jr., J. A. McLachlan, "Synergistic Activation of Estrogen Receptor with Combinations of Environmental Chemicals," *Science*, June 7, 1996, pp. 1489–92.

133. "'Environmental Estrogens' May Pose Greater Risk, Study Shows," *Washington Post,* June 7, 1996.

134. "Study Warns of Effects of Mixed Chemicals," *Los Angeles Times*, June 7, 1996.

135. K. Ramamoorthy, F. Wang, I. C. Chen, S. Safe, J. D. Norris, D. P. McDonnell, K. W. Gaido, W. Bocchinfuso, K. S. Korach, "Potency of Combined Estrogenic Pesticides," *Science*, January 17, 1997, pp. 405–6.

136. J. Ashby, P. A. Lefevre, J. Odum, C. A. Harris, E. J. Routledge, J. P. Sumpter, "Synergy between Synthetic Estrogens?" *Nature*, February 6, 1997, p. 494.

137. J. A. McLachlan, "Synergistic Effect of Environmental Estrogens: Report Withdrawn," *Science*, July 1997, pp. 462–63.

138. "Controversial Results of an Experiment Retracted," *Times-Picayune*, July 26, 1997.

139. "Tulane Researchers Retract Findings on Pollutants' Risk; University Begins Inquiry to 'Assure That Proper Laboratory Practices Were Followed,'" *Washington Post*, August 17, 1997.

140. R. T. Burkman, "Association between Intrauterine Device and Pelvic Inflammatory Disease," *Obstetrics and Gynecology,* March 1981, pp. 269–76.

141. "Study Challenges Federal Research on Risks of IUD's," *New York Times*, April 15, 1991.

142. R. A. Kronmal, C. W. Whitney, S. D. Mumford, "The Intrauterine Device and Pelvic Inflammatory Disease: The Women's Health Study Reanalyzed," *Journal of Clinical Epidemiology*, February 1991, pp. 109–22.

143. "American Home's 'Steal Deal' for A.H. Robins," *Washington Post*, December 15, 1989.

144. A. Ascherio, M. B. Katan, P. L. Zock, M. J. Stampfer, W. C. Willett, "Trans Fatty Acids and Coronary Heart Disease," *New England Journal of Medicine*, June 24, 1999, pp. 1994–98.

Lesson 3

145. "Medical Mistakes Blamed for Up to 98,000 Deaths a Year," *Fort Worth Star-Telegram*, November 30, 1999.

146. See, for example, "Clinton Wants Hospitals to Report Deadly Mistakes," Associated Press, February 22, 2000.

147. D. M. Lloyd-Jones, D. O. Martin, M. G. Larson, D. Levy, "Accuracy of Death Certificates for Coding Coronary Heart Disease as the Cause of Death," *Annals of Internal Medicine*, December 15, 1998, pp. 1020–26.

148. "Death-Certificate Study: CHD Deaths Overstated," *Medical Outcomes & Guidelines Alert*, December 17, 1998.

149. Ibid.

150. I. Kawachi, G. A. Colditz, F. E. Speizer, J. E. Manson, M. J. Stampfer, W. C. Willett, C. H. Hennekens, "A Prospective Study of Passive Smoking and Coronary Heart Disease," *Circulation*, May 20, 1997, pp. 2374–79.

151. W. D. Rosamond, J. M. Sprafka, P. G. McGovern, M. Nelson, R. V. Luepker, "Validation of Self-reported History of Acute Myocardial Infarction: Experience of the Minnesota Heart Survey Registry," *Epidemiology*, January 6, 1995, pp. 67–69.

152. A. J. Wells, P. B. English, S. F. Posner, L. E. Wagenknecht, E. J. Perez-Stable, "Misclassification Rates for Current Smokers Misclassified as Nonsmokers," *American Journal of Public Health*, October 1998, pp. 1503–9.

153. B. M. Rifkind, J. E. Rossouw, "Of Designer Drugs, Magic Bullets, and Gold Standards," *Journal of the American Medical Association*, May 13, 1998, pp. 1483–85.

154. "Smoking Is Too Often a Child's Decision," *St. Petersburg Times*, August 5, 1990.

155. J. P. Pierce, M. C. Fiore, T. E. Novotny, E. J. Hatziandreu, R. M. Davis, "Trends in Cigarette Smoking in the United States: Projections to the Year 2000," *Journal of the American Medical Association*, January 6, 1989, pp. 61–65.

156. A recent study from the CDC used a confusing statistical analysis to conveniently arrive at the 3,000 estimate, supposedly affirming the statistic.

157. Jews for the Preservation of Firearms, "HCI Conceals Data to Mislead President, Press and Public on Child Deaths, Says Gun Advocacy Group," U.S. Newswire, March 6, 2000.

158. This figure was subsequently reduced to 15,000 when it was pointed out that the EPA made an elementary statistical error. See "EPA Concedes Error in Air Pollution Claim; Estimate of Lives Saved by New Rules Is Lowered," *Washington Post*, April 3, 1997.

159. B. G. Charlton, "Statistical Malpractice," *Journal of the Royal College of Physicians in London*, March–April, 1996, pp. 112–14.

160. National Research Council, *Possible Health Effects of Exposure to Residential Electric and Magnetic Fields* (Washington: National Academy Press, 1996).

161. "Agent Orange and Diabetes: Diving into Murky Depths," *New York Times*, March 30, 2000.

162. See, for example, M. P. Longnecker, J. E. Michalek, "Serum Dioxin Level in Relation to Diabetes Mellitus among Air Force Veterans with Background Levels of Exposure," *Epidemi-*

ology, January 2000, pp. 44–48; G. M. Calvert, M. H. Sweeney, J. Deddens, D. K. Wall, "Evaluation of Diabetes Mellitus, Serum Glucose, and Thyroid Function among United States Workers Exposed to 2,3,7,8-Tetrachlorodibenzo-p-dioxin," *Journal of Occupational and Environmental Medicine*, April, 1999, pp. 270–76; K. Steenland, L. Piacitelli, J. Deddens, M. Fingerhut, L. I. Chang, "Cancer, Heart Disease, and Diabetes in Workers Exposed to 2,3,7,8-Tetrachlorodibenzo-p-dioxin," *Journal of the National Cancer Institute*, May 5, 1999, pp. 779–86; A. C. Pesatori, C. Zocchetti, S. Guercilena, D. Consonni, D. Turrini, P. A. Bertazzi, "Dioxin Exposure and Non-malignant Health Effects: A Mortality Study," *Journal of Occupational and Environmental Medicine*, February 1998, pp. 126–33; J. Vena, P. Boffetta, H. Becher, T. Benn, H. B. Bueno-de-Mesquita, D. Coggon, D. Colin, D. Flesch-Janys, L. Green, T. Kauppinen, M. Littorin, E. Lynge, J. D. Mathews, M. Neuberger, N. Pearce, A. C. Pesatori, R. Saracci, K. Steenland, M. Kogevinas, "Exposure to Dioxin and Non-neoplastic Mortality in the Expanded IARC International Cohort Study of Phenoxy Herbicide and Chlorophenol Production Workers and Sprayers," *Environmental Health Perspectives*, April 1998, pp. 645–53.

163. M. D. Eisner, A. K. Smith, P. D. Blanc, "Bartenders' Respiratory Health after Establishment of Smoke-free Bars and Taverns," *Journal of the American Medical Association*, December 9, 1998, pp. 1909–14.

164. Ibid.

165. Charlton.

166. D. A. Leon, "Failed or Misleading Adjustment for Confounding," *Lancet*, August 21, 1993, pp. 479–81.

167. "Second-hand Smoke Linked to Breast Cancer," *Toronto Star*, March 16, 2000.

168. See K. C. Johnson, J. Hu, Y. Mao, "Passive and Active Smoking and Breast Cancer Risk in Canada, 1994–97," *Cancer Causes and Control*, March 2000, pp. 211–21.

169. See, for example, J. Verloop, M. A. Rookus, K. van der Kooy, F. E. van Leeuwen, "Physical Activity and Breast Cancer Risk in Women Aged 20–54 years," *Journal of the National Cancer Institute*, January 19, 2000, pp. 128–35; L. Velie, M. Kulldorff, C. Schairer, G. Block, D. Albanes, A. Schatzkin, "Dietary Fat, Fat Subtypes, and Breast Cancer in Postmenopausal Women: A Prospective Cohort Study," *Journal of the National Cancer Institute*, May 17, 2000, pp. 833–39.

170. See K. Armstrong, A. Eisen, B. Weber, "Assessing the Risk of Breast Cancer," *New England Journal of Medicine*, February 24, 2000, pp. 564–71.

171. See, for example, G. A. Colditz, "Hormone Replacement Therapy Increases the Risk of Breast Cancer," *Annals of the New York Academy of Sciences*, December 29, 1997, pp. 129–36.

Lesson 4

172. D. E. Lilienfeld and P. D. Stolley. *Foundations of Epidemiology*, 3d ed. (New York: Oxford University Press, 1994).

173. See S. R. Cummings, S. Eckert, K. A. Krueger, D. Grady, T. J. Powles, J. A. Cauley, L. Norton, T. Nickelsen, N. H. Bjarnason, M. Morrow, M. E. Lippman, D. Black, J. E. Glusman, A. Costa, V. C. Jordan, "The Effect of Raloxifene on Risk of Breast Cancer in Postmenopausal Women: Results from the MORE Randomized Trial; Multiple Outcomes of Raloxifene Evaluation," *Journal of the American Medical Association*. June 16, 1999, pp. 2189–97.

174. See G. W. Ross, R. D. Abbott, H. Petrovitch, D. M. Morens, A. Grandinetti, K. H. Tung, C. M. Tanner, K. H. Masaki, P. L. Blanchette, J. D. Curb, J. S. Popper, L. R. White,

"Association of Coffee and Caffeine Intake with the Risk of Parkinson's Disease," *Journal of the American Medical Association*, May 24, 2000, pp. 2674–79.

175. Z. F. Zhang, H. Morgenstern, M. R. Spitz, D. P. Tashkin, G. Yu, T. C. Hsu, S. Schantz, "Environmental Tobacco Smoking, Mutagen Sensitivity, and Head and Neck Squamous Cell Carcinoma," *Cancer Epidemiology, Biomarkers and Prevention*, 2000, pp. 1043–49.

176. W. G. Christen, U. A. Ajani, R. J. Glynn, C. H. Hennekens, "Blood Levels of Homocysteine and Increased Risks of Cardiovascular Disease: Causal or Casual?" *Archives of Internal Medicine*, February 28, 2000, pp. 422–34.

177. See D. M. Schreinemachers, "Cancer Mortality in Four Northern Wheat-producing States," *Environmental Health Perspectives*, September 2000, pp. 873–81.

178. D. W. Dockery, C. A. Pope III, X. Xu, J. D. Spengler, J. H. Ware, M. E. Fay, B. G. Ferris Jr., F. E. Speizer, "An Association between Air Pollution and Mortality in Six U.S. Cities," *New England Journal of Medicine*, December 9, 1993, pp. 1753–59.

179. P. Skrabanek, "The Emptiness of the Black Box," *Epidemiology*, September 5, 1994, pp. 553–55.

180. "New Study Says Women May Reduce Risk of Breast Cancer If They Exercise One Hour a Day," *NBA Today*, October 26, 1999.

181. B. Rockhill, W. C. Willett, D. J. Hunter, J. E. Manson, S. E. Hankinson, G. A. Colditz, "A Prospective Study of Recreational Physical Activity and Breast Cancer Risk," *Archives of Internal Medicine*, October 25, 1999, pp. 2290–96.

182. Ibid.

Lesson 5

183. E. L. Wynder, "Workshop on Guidelines to the Epidemiology of Weak Associations," *Preventive Medicine*, 1987, pp. 139–41.

184. A. B. Hill, "President's Address: Observed Association to a Verdict of Causation: Upon What Basis Should We Proceed to Do So?" *Proceedings of the Royal Society of Medicine*, 1968.

185. E. Wynder, "Epidemiology Faces Its Limits," *American Journal of Epidemiology*, 1996, pp. 747–49.

186. J. Brind, V. M. Chinchilli, W. B. Severs, J. Summy-Long, "Induced Abortion as an Independent Risk Factor for Breast Cancer: A Comprehensive Review and Meta-analysis," *Journal of Epidemiology and Community Health*, October 1996, pp. 481–96.

187. National Cancer Institute, "Abortion and Possible Risk for Breast Cancer: Analysis and Inconsistencies," October 26, 1994.

188. "Review of 23 Studies Links Abortion and Breast Cancer," *Washington Post*, October 12, 1996.

189. "Study on Abortion and Cancer Spurs Fight—Claims about a Higher Risk of Breast Disease Spill into Subways and Courts," *Wall Street Journal*, October 11, 1996.

Lesson 6

190. M. Gronbaek, U. Becker, D. Johansen, A. Gottschau, P. Schnohr, H. O. Hein, G. Jensen, T. I. Sorensen, "Type of Alcohol Consumed and Mortality from All Causes, Coronary Heart Disease, and Cancer," *Annals of Internal Medicine*, September 19, 2000, pp. 411–19.

191. F. D. Gilliland, W. C. Hunt, V. E. Archer, G. Saccomanno, "Radon Progeny Exposure and Lung Cancer Risk among Non-smoking Uranium Miners," *Health Physics*, October 2000, pp. 365–72.

192. P. Boffetta, J. Tredaniel, A. Greco. "Risk of Childhood Cancer and Adult Lung Cancer after Childhood Exposure to Passive Smoke: A Meta-analysis," *Environmental Health Perspectives*, January 2000, pp. 73–82.

193. Gronbaek et al.

194. D. B. Moore, A. R. Folsom, P. J. Mink, C. P. Hong, K. E. Anderson, L. H. Kushi, "Physical Activity and Incidence of Postmenopausal Breast Cancer," *Epidemiology*, May 2000, pp. 292–96.

195. *Armstrong v. Osteen*, No. 01-1299, No. 01-1300, U.S. Court of Appeals for the Fourth Circuit, April 20, 2001.

196. Gilliland et al.

197. Gronbaek et al.

Lesson 7

198. J. P. Kassirer, M. Angell, "Losing Weight—An Ill-fated New Year's Resolution," *New England Journal of Medicine*, January 1, 1998, pp. 52–54.

199. J. P. Kassirer, M. Angell, "The Obesity Problem," *New England Journal of Medicine*, April 1998, p. 1158.

200. L. S. Miller, X. Zhang, D. P. Rice, W. Max, "State Estimates of Total Medical Expenditures Attributable to Cigarette Smoking, 1993," *Public Health Reports*, September–October 1998, pp. 447–58.

Lesson 8

201. International Agency for Research on Cancer, Monograph 73 (1999), p. 517.

202. Environmental Working Group, "Government Underestimates Infant Exposure to Toxic Weed Killer," July 28, 1999.

203. International Agency for Research on Cancer, p. 59.

204. For a full discussion, see Regulatory Impact Analysis Project, "Choices in Risk Assessment: The Role of Science Policy in the Environmental Risk Management Process," RIAP, Washington, 1994.

205. P. H. Abelson, "Diet and Cancer in Humans and Rodents," *Science*, January 10, 1992, p. 141.

206. P. H. Abelson, "Flaws in Risk Assessments," *Science*, October 13, 1995, p. 215.

207. R. D. Kimbrough, R. A. Squire, R. E. Linder, J. D. Strandberg, R. J. Montalli, V. W. Burse, "Induction of Liver Tumor in Sherman Strain Female Rats by Polychlorinated Biphenyl Aroclor 1260," *Journal of the National Cancer Institute*, December, 1975, pp. 1453–59.

208. "The New War on Cancer—Carter Team Seeks Causes, Not Cures," *National Journal*, August 6, 1977.

209. R. D. Kimbrough, M. L. Doemland, M. E. LeVois, "Mortality in Male and Female Capacitor Workers Exposed to Polychlorinated Biphenyls," *Journal of Occupational and Environmental Medicine*, March 1999, pp. 161–71.

210. See G. S. Cooper, M. P. Longnecker, D. P. Sandler, R. B. Ness, "Risk of Ovarian Cancer in Relation to Use of Phenolphthalein-containing Laxatives," *British Journal of Cancer*, August 2000, pp. 404–6; M. P. Longnecker, D. P. Sandler, R. W. Haile, R. S. Sandler, "Phenolphthalein-containing Laxative Use in Relation to Adenomatous Colorectal Polyps in Three Studies," *Environmental Health Perspectives*, November 1997, pp. 1210–12; G. A. Kune, "Laxative Use Not a Risk for Colorectal Cancer: Data from the Melbourne Colorectal Cancer Study," *Zeitschrift für Gastroenterologie*, February 1993, pp. 140–43.

211. "Dioxin Can Harm Tooth Development," *Science News*, February 20, 1999.

212. S. Alaluusua, P. L. Lukinmaa, R. Pohjanvirta, M. Unkila, J. Tuomisto, "Exposure to 2,3,7,8-Tetrachlorodibenzo-para-dioxin Leads to Defective Dentin Formation and Pulpal Perforation in Rat Incisor Tooth," *Toxicology*, July 11, 1993, pp. 1–13.

213. *New York Times*, February 4, 1976.

214. "Consumer Group Links Caffeine with Birth Defects," Associated Press, November 19, 1979.

215. "FDA to Warn On Caffeine in Pregnancy," *Washington Post*, September 4, 1980.

216. Ibid.

217. Center for Science in the Public Interest, "Label Caffeine Content of Foods, Scientists Tell FDA; Health Activists Say Caffeine Causes More Than a 'Buzz': Miscarriages, Withdrawal Symptoms, Poor Nutrition," July 31, 1997.

218. K. S. Crump, D. Krewski, C. Van Landingham, "Estimates of the Proportion of Chemicals That Were Carcinogenic or Anticarcinogenic in Bioassays Conducted by the National Toxicology Program," *Environmental Health Perspectives*, 1999, pp. 83–88.

Lesson 9

219. Dr. Marilie Gammon, a Columbia University statistician who is a principal investigator for a study, mandated by Congress and administered by the National Cancer Institute, which is part of the U.S. Department of Health and Human Services, to look into the Long Island cancer rates, cited in "Findings Don't Account for Long Island's High Cancer Rate," *New York Times*, September 29, 1995.

220. "EPA Links Dioxin to Cancer; Risk Estimate Raised Tenfold," *Washington Post*, May 17, 2000.

221. M. Gough, S. Milloy, "CALUX™ and GC/MS Analysis of TEQ Contamination for Risk Assessment of Exposure to Dioxins in Ice Cream," *Proceedings of the 20th International Symposium on Halogenated Environmental Organic Pollutants & POPS*, 2000, pp. 320–23.

Lesson 10

222. C. M. Mahan, T. A. Bullman, H. K. Kang, S. Selvin, "A Case-control Study of Lung Cancer among Vietnam Veterans," *Journal of Occupational and Environmental Medicine*, August 1997, pp. 740–47.

223. M. C. Ha, S. Cordier, D. Bard, T. B. Le, A. H. Hoang, T. Q. Hoang, C. D. Le, L. Abenhaim, T. N. Nguyen, "Agent Orange and the Risk of Gestational Trophoblastic Disease in Vietnam," *Archives of Environmental Health*, September–October 1996, pp. 368–74.

224. N. A. Dalager, H. K. Kang, V. L. Burt, L. Weatherbee, "Hodgkin's Disease and Vietnam Service," *Annals of Epidemiology*, September 1995, pp. 400–406.

225. N. A. Dalager, H. K. Kang, V. L. Burt, L. Weatherbee, "Non-Hodgkin's Lymphoma among Vietnam Veterans," *Journal of Occupational Medicine*, July 1991, pp. 774–79.

226. Selected Cancers Cooperative Study Group, "The Association of Selected Cancers with Service in the US Military in Vietnam, III: Hodgkin's Disease, Nasal Cancer, Nasopharyngeal Cancer, and Primary Liver Cancer," *Archives of Internal Medicine*, December 1990, pp. 2495–505.

227. W. H. Wolfe, J. E. Michalek, J. C. Miner, A. Rahe, J. Silva, W. F. Thomas, W. D. Grubbs, M. B. Lustik, T. G. Karrison, R. H. Roegner, et al., "Health Status of Air Force Veterans Occupationally Exposed to Herbicides in Vietnam, I: Physical Health," *Journal of the American Medical Association*, October 1990, pp. 1824–31.

228. G. C. Caldwell, "Twenty-two Years of Cancer Cluster Investigations at the Centers for Disease Control," *American Journal of Epidemiology*, July 1990, pp. S43–47.

229. Ibid.

230. C. W. Trumbo, "Public Requests for Cancer Cluster Investigations: A Survey of State Health Departments," *American Journal of Public Health*, August 2000, pp. 1300–302.

231. N. Cobb. "Investigating Cancer Clusters," *International Journal of Circumpolar Health*, 1998, pp. 27–30.

232. C. W. Heath Jr., "Investigating Causation in Cancer Clusters," *Radiation and Environmental Biophysics*, August 1996, pp. 133–36.

233. "Controversial Estimate of Chernobyl-Linked Cancers," Associated Press, September 9, 1986.

234. "Chernobyl 'Not So Deadly,'" British Broadcasting Corporation, June 13, 2000.

235. "Chernobyl Radiation Stirs Quick Mutation in Plants," Associated Press, October 4, 2000.

236. U.S. Environmental Protection Agency, *1998 Children's Environmental Health Yearbook*.

237. S. Grufferman, "Methodologic Approaches to Studying Environmental Factors in Childhood Cancer," *Environmental Health Perspectives*, June 1998, pp. 881–86.

238. "Cancer in Children under 15," *Journal of the National Cancer Institute*, 1999, p. 503.

239. M. S. Linet, L. A. Ries, M. A. Smith, R. E. Tarone, S. S. Devesa, "Cancer Surveillance Series: Recent Trends in Childhood Cancer Incidence and Mortality in the United States," *Journal of the National Cancer Institute*, June 1999, pp. 1051–58.

240. M. A. Smith, B. Freidlin, L. A. Ries, R. Simon, "Trends in Reported Incidence of Primary Malignant Brain Tumors in Children in the United States," *Journal of the National Cancer Institute*, September 1998, pp. 1269–77.

241. C. La Vecchia, F. Levi, F. Lucchini, P. Lagiou, D. Trichopoulos, E. Negri, "Trends in Childhood Cancer Mortality as Indicators of the Quality of Medical Care in the Developed World," *Cancer*, November 1998, pp. 2,223–27.

242. U.S. Environmental Protection Agency, "Childhood Cancer," Office of Children's Health Protection, http://www.epa.gov/children/cancer.htm.

243. See, for example, M. Steinbuch, C. R. Weinberg, J. D. Buckley, L. L. Robison, D. P. Sandler, "Indoor Residential Radon Exposure and Risk of Childhood Acute Myeloid Leukemia," *British Journal of Cancer*, November 1999, pp. 900–906.

244. U. Kaletsch, P. Kaatsch, R. Meinert, J. Schuz, R. Czarwinski, J. Michaelis, "Childhood Cancer and Residential Radon Exposure—Results of a Population-based Case-control Study

in Lower Saxony (Germany)," *Radiation and Environmental Biophysics*, September 1999, pp. 211–15.

245. S. P. Cooper, A. E. Fraire, P. A. Buffler, S. D. Greenberg, C. Langston, "Epidemiologic Aspects of Childhood Mesothelioma," *Pathology and Immunopathology Research*, August 1989, pp. 276–86.

246. See, for example, S. J. Orlow, "Melanomas in Children," *Pediatrics in Review*, October 1995, pp. 365–69; B. W. LeSueur, N. G. Silvis, R. C. Hansen, "Basal Cell Carcinoma in Children: Report of 3 Cases," *Archives of Dermatology*, March 2000, pp. 370–72.

247. D. B. Buller, R. Borland, "Skin Cancer Prevention for Children: A Critical Review," *Health, Education and Behavior*, June 1999, pp. 317–43.

248. E. White, T. E. Aldrich, "Geographic Studies of Pediatric Cancer Near Hazardous Waste Sites," *Archives of Environmental Health*, November–December 1999, pp. 390–97.

249. E. Knox, "Childhood Cancers, Birthplaces, Incinerators and Landfill Sites," *International Journal of Epidemiology*, June 2000, pp. 391–97.

250. J. L. Daniels, A. F. Olshan, D. A. Savitz, "Pesticides and Childhood Cancers," *Environmental Health Perspectives*, October 1997, pp. 1068–77.

251. See, for example, "EPA Bans Popular Pesticide; Valley Tree-Fruit Farmers Must Scramble to Find a Replacement," *Fresno Bee*, August 3, 1999.

252. G. Ostergaard, I. Knudsen, "The Applicability of the ADI (Acceptable Daily Intake) for Food Additives to Infants and Children," *Food Additives and Contaminants*, 1998, pp. S63–74.

253. A. G. Renwick, "Toxicokinetics in Infants and Children in Relation to the ADI and TDI," *Food Additives and Contaminants*, 1998, pp. S17–35.

254. C. Steinberg, C. A. Notterman, "Pharmacokinetics of Cardiovascular Drugs in Children: Inotropes and Vasopressors," *Clinical Pharmacokinetics*, November 1994, pp. 345–67.

255. J. V. Aranda, J. M. Collinge, R. Zinman, G. Watters, "Maturation of Caffeine Elimination in Infancy," *Archives of Diseases in Children*, December 1979, pp. 946–49.

256. R. Carson, *Silent Spring* (New York: Houghton Mifflin, 1962).

257. See, for example, S. Takayama, S. M. Sieber, D. W. Dalgard, U. P. Thorgeirsson, R. H. Adamson, "Effects of Long-term Oral Administration of DDT on Nonhuman Primates," *Journal of Cancer Research and Clinical Oncology*, 1999, pp. 219–25; K. J. Helzlsouer, A. J. Alberg, H. Y. Huang, S. C. Hoffman, P. T. Strickland, J. W. Brock, W. V. Burse, L. L. Needham, D. A. Bell, J. A. Lavigne, J. D. Yager, G. W. Comstock, "Serum Concentrations of Organochlorine Compounds and the Subsequent Development of Breast Cancer," *Cancer Epidemiology Biomarkers and Prevention*, June 1999, pp. 525–32; J. F. Dorgan, J. W. Brock, N. Rothman, L. L. Needham, R. Miller, H. E. Stephenson Jr., N. Schussler, P. R. Taylor, "Serum Organochlorine Pesticides and PCBs and Breast Cancer Risk: Results from a Prospective Analysis (USA)," *Cancer Causes and Control*, February 1999, pp. 1–11; D. Baris, S. H. Zahm, K. P. Cantor, A. Blair, "Agricultural Use of DDT and Risk of Non-Hodgkin's Lymphoma: Pooled Analysis of Three Case-control Studies in the United States," *Journal of Occupational and Environmental Medicine*, August 1998, pp. 522–27; D. J. Hunter, S. E. Hankinson, F. Laden, G. A. Colditz, J. E. Manson, W. C. Willett, F. E. Speizer, M. S. Wolff, "Plasma Organochlorine Levels and the Risk of Breast Cancer," *New England Journal of Medicine*, October 1997, pp. 1253–58; P. van't Veer, I. E. Lobbezoo, J. M. Martin-Moreno, E. Guallar, J. Gomez-Aracena, A. F. Kardinaal, L. Kohlmeier, B. C. Martin, J. J. Strain, M. Thamm, P. van Zoonen, B. A. Baumann, J. K. Huttunen, F. J. Kok, "DDT (Dicophane) and Postmenopausal

Breast Cancer in Europe: Case-control Study," *British Medical Journal*, July 1997, pp. 81–85; J. Higginson, *DDT: Epidemiological Evidence* (Lyon, France: International Agency for Research on Cancer Scientific Publications, 1985), pp. 107–17; J. R. Cabral, R. K. Hall, L. Rossi, S. A. Bronczyk, P. Shubik, "Lack of Carcinogenicity of DDT in Hamsters," *Tumori*, February 1982, pp. 5–10; K. C. Silinskas, A. B. Okey, "Protection by 1,1,1-trichloro-2,2-bis(p-chloro-phenyl)ethane (DDT) against Mammary Tumors and Leukemia during Prolonged Feeding of 7,12-dimethylbenz(a)anthracene to Female Rats," *Journal of the National Cancer Institute*, September 1975, pp. 653–57.

258. E. M. Sweeney, "EPA Hearing Examiner's Recommendations and Findings Concerning DDT Hearings," April 25, 1972.

259. S. J. Milloy, "100 Things You Should Know about DDT," 1999, http://www.junkscience.com/ddtfaq.html.

260. C. Ernhart, S. Scarr, D. F. Geneson, "On Being a Whistleblower: The Needleman Case," *Ethics and Behavior*, 1993, pp. 73–93.

261. Ibid., pp. 77–78.

262. U.S. Environmental Protection Agency, "Independent Peer Review of Selected Studies Concerned Neurobehavioral Effects of Lead Exposures in Nominally Asymptomatic Children: Official Report of Findings and Recommendations of an Interdisciplinary Expert Review Committee," EPA-600/8-83-028A, 1983.

263. Needleman Inquiry Panel, *Needleman Inquiry Final Report* (Pittsburgh: University of Pittsburgh, 1991).

264. E. J. Schoen, "Blood Lead Levels, Scientific Misconduct and the Needleman Case, 2: The Critics' Arguments," *New England Journal of Medicine*, January 1996, pp. 112–13.

265. S. J. Pocock, M. Smith, P. Baghurst, "Environmental Lead and Children's Intelligence: A Systematic Review of the Epidemiological Evidence," *British Medical Journal*, November 1994, pp. 1189–97.

266. Jane See White, Niagara Falls, N.Y., Associated Press, August 3, 1978.

267. E. Whelan, *Toxic Terror*, 2d ed. (Buffalo, N.Y.: Prometheus Books, 1993), pp. 125–29.

268. P. H. Abelson, "Chemicals from Waste Dumps," *Science*, July 26, 1985, p. 335.

269. N. J. Vianna, A. K. Polan, "Incidence of Low Birth Weight among Love Canal Residents," *Science*, December 7, 1984, pp. 1217–19.

270. Ibid.

271. C. W. Heath Jr., M. R. Nadel, M. M. Zack Jr., A. T. Chen, M. A. Bender, R. J. Preston, "Cytogenetic Findings in Persons Living Near the Love Canal," *Journal of the American Medical Association*, March 16, 1984, pp. 1437–40.

272. D. T. Janerich, W. S. Burnett, G. Feck, M. Hoff, P. Nasca, A. P. Polednak, P. Greenwald, N. Vianna, "Cancer Incidence in the Love Canal Area," *Science*, June 19, 1981, pp. 1404–7.

273. "Buck Often Stops at Top in Accidents; Oversight a Key Issue, Bonfire Investigators Says [sic]," *Dallas Morning News*, January 19, 2000; ABC News, *World News Tonight*, April 28, 2000.

274. E. O. Talbott, A. O. Youk, K. P. McHugh, J. D. Shire, A. Zhang, B. P. Murphy, R. A. Engberg, "Mortality among the Residents of the Three Mile Island Accident Area: 1979–1992," *Environmental Health Perspectives*, June 2000, pp. 545–52.

Lesson 11

275. See Indur M. Goklany, *The Precautionary Principle: A Critical Appraisal of Environmental Risk Assessment* (Washington: Cato Institute, October 2001).

276. "Study: No Link between Hanford Radiation Releases and Thyroid Disease," Associated Press, January 29, 1999.

277. "Federal Panel: Earlier Study Overstated Little Risk for Thyroid Disease" Associated Press, December 15, 1999.

278. "EU/WTO: Seattle Delegates Grind through Painful Agenda," *European Report*, December 4, 1999.

279. "Secondhand Smoke Peril Affirmed; EPA Move to Endorse Report on Cigarettes May Affect Workplace," *Washington Post*, January 6, 1993.

280. "EPA to Declare Passive Smoke Causes Cancer," *Los Angeles Times*, January 6, 1993.

281. J. He, S. Vupputuri, K. Allen, M. R. Prerost, J. Hughes, P. K. Whelton, "Passive Smoking and the Risk of Coronary Heart Disease—A Meta-analysis of Epidemiologic Studies," *New England Journal of Medicine*, March 25, 1999, pp. 920–26.

282. J. D. Bailar III, "Passive Smoking, Coronary Heart Disease, and Meta-analysis," *New England Journal of Medicine*, March 25, 1999, pp. 958–59.

283. "Handgun Control Inc.: After Shootings, Gun Lobby and GOP Candidates Try to Talk the Talk about Guns," U.S. Newswire, March 3, 2000.

284. S. P. Teret, D. W. Webster, "Reducing Gun Deaths in the United States," *British Medical Journal*, May 1, 1999, pp. 1160–61.

285. Adapted from K. Steenland, L. Piacitelli, J. Deddens, M. Fingerhut, L. I. Chang, "Cancer, Heart Disease, and Diabetes in Workers Exposed to 2,3,7,8-tetrachlorodibenzo-p-dioxin," *Journal of the National Cancer Institute*, May 5, 1999, pp. 779–86.

286. "High Selenium Levels May Ward Off Cancer," *Los Angeles Times*, August 19, 1998.

287. K. Yoshizawa, W. C. Willett, S. J. Morris, M. J. Stampfer, D. Spiegelman, E. B. Rimm, E. Giovannucci, "Study of Prediagnostic Selenium Level in Toenails and the Risk of Advanced Prostate Cancer," *Journal of the National Cancer Institute*, August 19, 1998, pp. 1219–24.

288. F. B. Hu, M. J. Stampfer, J. E. Manson, E. Rimm, G. A. Colditz, B. A. Rosner, C. H. Hennekens, W. C. Willett, "Dietary Fat Intake and the Risk of Coronary Heart Disease in Women," *New England Journal of Medicine*, November 20, 1997, pp. 1491–99.

289. See A. P. Hoyer, P. Grandjean, T. Jorgensen, J. W. Brock, H. B. Hartvig, "Organochlorine Exposure and Risk of Breast Cancer," *Lancet*, December 5, 1998, pp. 1816–20.

290. R. C. Brownson, M. C. Alavanja, E. T. Hock, T. S. Loy, "Passive Smoking and Lung Cancer in Nonsmoking Women," *American Journal of Public Health*, November 1992, pp. 1525–30.

291. "Risk Studies Differ on Passive Smoking," *Washington Times*, November 20, 1992.

292. Environmental Working Group, "One Million Kids a Day Exposed to Unsafe Levels of Toxic Pesticides in Fruit, Vegetables, and Baby Food; Report Urges Ban on Dangerous Insecticides," January 29, 1998.

293. Environmental Working Group, "Tough to Swallow: How Pesticide Companies Profit from Poisoning America's Tap Water," Media release, August 12, 1997.

294. "Groups Debate Water Standards," *Columbus Dispatch*, August 13, 1997.

295. See http://www.cs.virginia.edu/oracle/bacon_info.html.

296. M. E. J. Newman, "The Structure of Scientific Collaboration Networks, *Proceedings of the National Academy of Sciences*, January 16, 2001, pp. 404–09.

297. "Quality Control of Published Medical Studies Debated," *Washington Post*, May 14, 1989.

298. U.S. House of Representatives, Committee on Government Reform, "Exposure to Hazardous Air Pollutants in Los Angeles (Minority Report)," March 1, 1999.

299. "Harvard Study Finds No Evidence of Connection between Dietary Fat Intake and Incidence of Breast Cancer," CBS News Transcripts, March 9, 1999.

300. A. H. Wu, M. C. Pike, D. O. Stram, "Meta-analysis: Dietary Fat Intake, Serum Estrogen Levels, and the Risk of Breast Cancer,"*Journal of the National Cancer Institute*, March 17, 1999, pp. 529–34.

301. Ibid.

302. "Smokers' Sons More Violent, Study Says," *Los Angeles Times*, March 15, 1999.

303. D. M. Fergusson, "Prenatal Smoking and Antisocial Behavior,"*Archives of General Psychiatry*, March 1999, pp. 223–24.

304. J. Lowy, "Favored Home Insecticide to Be Deemed Unsafe," Scripps Howard News Service, May 24, 2000.

305. "Widely Used Pesticide May Be More of a Health Risk Than Previously Thought," *CBS Evening News*, June 1, 2000.

306. E. Wong, "In New York's War on Bugs, a Call for New Ammunition," *New York Times*, June 9, 2000.

307. "Some Chemical Solvents Found In Work Environments May Pose Risks to Pregnant Women," CBS News Transcripts, March 24, 1999.

308. S. Khattak, G. K-Moghtader, K. McMartin, M. Barrera, D. Kennedy, G. Koren, "Pregnancy Outcome Following Gestational Exposure to Organic Solvents: A Prospective Controlled Study," *Journal of the American Medical Association*, March 24–31, 1999, pp. 1106–9.

309. K. I. McMartin, M. Chu, E. Kopecky, T. R. Einarson, G. Koren, "Pregnancy Outcome Following Maternal Organic Solvent Exposure: A Meta-analysis of Epidemiologic Studies," *American Journal of Industrial Medicine*, September 1998, pp. 288–92.

A Final Word

310. 5 U.S.C. §706(2)(A).

311. See *Chevron U.S.A. v. Natural Resources Defense Council*, 467 U.S. 837 (1984).

312. *AFL-CIO v. OSHA*, 965 F.2d 962 (11th Cir. 1992).

313. *Daubert v. Merrell Dow Pharm., Inc.*, 509 U.S. 579 (1993).

314. W. Piermattei, "From *Frye* to *Joiner*: The Supreme Court Muddies the Waters of Judicial Reasoning," *Vermont's Journal of the Environment*, 1999, http://www.vje.org.

INDEX

ABOUT THE AUTHOR

Steven J. Milloy is the publisher of JunkScience.com, an adjunct scholar at the Cato Institute, and a columnist for FoxNews.com.

JunkScience.com has garnered numerous awards, including being named a "Top Resource" by Yahoo!, "One of the 50 Best Web Sites of 1998" by *Popular Science*, and a "Hot Pick" by *Science*. Junk science.com has also been spotlighted by the *Washington Post*, the *New York Times*, the *Los Angeles Times*, *USA Today*, the *Detroit News*, the *Times* (UK), the *Financial Times*, *Forbes*, MSNBC, and many other popular media outlets.

Milloy has published more than 100 newspaper and magazine articles on junk science issues, appears frequently on radio and television, has testified on risk assessment and Superfund before the U.S. Congress, and has lectured before numerous organizations.

Other books written by Milloy include *Science without Sense* (Cato Institute, 1995) and *Science-Based Risk Assessment: A Piece of the Superfund Puzzle* (National Environmental Policy Institute, 1995). He coauthored with Dr. Michael Gough *Silencing Science* (Cato Institute, 1999).

Milloy holds a B.A. in natural sciences from the Johns Hopkins University, a master of health sciences in biostatistics from the Johns Hopkins University School of Hygiene and Public Health, a juris doctorate from the University of Baltimore, and a master of laws from the Georgetown University Law Center.

Cato Institute

Founded in 1977, the Cato Institute is a public policy research foundation dedicated to broadening the parameters of policy debate to allow consideration of more options that are consistent with the traditional American principles of limited government, individual liberty, and peace. To that end, the Institute strives to achieve greater involvement of the intelligent, concerned lay public in questions of policy and the proper role of government.

The Institute is named for *Cato's Letters,* libertarian pamphlets that were widely read in the American Colonies in the early 18th century and played a major role in laying the philosophical foundation for the American Revolution.

Despite the achievement of the nation's Founders, today virtually no aspect of life is free from government encroachment. A pervasive intolerance for individual rights is shown by government's arbitrary intrusions into private economic transactions and its disregard for civil liberties.

To counter that trend, the Cato Institute undertakes an extensive publications program that addresses the complete spectrum of policy issues. Books, monographs, and shorter studies are commissioned to examine the federal budget, Social Security, regulation, military spending, international trade, and myriad other issues. Major policy conferences are held throughout the year, from which papers are published thrice yearly in the *Cato Journal.* The Institute also publishes the quarterly magazine *Regulation.*

In order to maintain its independence, the Cato Institute accepts no government funding. Contributions are received from foundations, corporations, and individuals, and other revenue is generated from the sale of publications. The Institute is a nonprofit, tax-exempt, educational foundation under Section 501(c)3 of the Internal Revenue Code.

CATO INSTITUTE
1000 Massachusetts Ave., N.W.
Washington, D.C. 20001